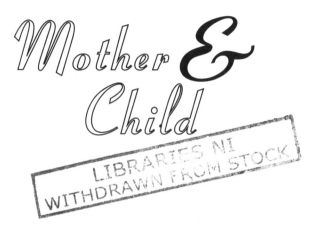

Mother & Child

Jan de Vries

D1610507

MAINSTREAM
PUBLISHING

EDINBURGH AND LONDON

First published in Great Britain in 2002 by
MAINSTREAM PUBLISHING COMPANY (EDINBURGH) LTD
7 Albany Street
Edinburgh EH1 3UG

ISBN 1 84018 428 0

A catalogue record for this book is available from the British Library

Typeset in Garamond
Printed and bound in Great Britain by
Cox & Wyman Ltd

Contents

Introduction

*M*other and Child* is not like other books on the subject of childcare. It is a practical approach to the best way to care for children growing up in a world full of pollution and other influences that may adversely affect their health, mentally, emotionally and physically. As a father and grandfather of four children and ten grandchildren, I have some experience of this! I have also taken care of both adults and children as patients for nearly 45 years and have given some of my findings in this book.

When writing *Mother and Child*, I asked my youngest daughter Maria, and her husband, Marcus, who have three wonderful, healthy boys, to pass on some of their advice, based on their experience of bringing up children in the 21st century. In this rapidly changing world, adjustments have to be made in how we look after our children. It is a great privilege to have them, but we also have a great responsibility from the time we bring them into this world until they grow up and want to stand on their own feet. Children are only 'lent material' and one day they will have to look after themselves. We can only, for as long as they are entrusted to us, do the very best for them.

I am sure that the knowledge passed on by Maria and Marcus in this book will be of help in filling the gaps in other books on this subject. I do hope that it will find its way into many homes, where we can share the experience of looking after our little treasures to the best of our ability.

ONE

Nature or Nurture?

Whilst I was thinking of writing this book – which I had put off for quite some time – something happened which inspired me to start it. After a very busy day at my practice in Montagu Street in London, I rushed to get a train from Liverpool Street station to Stansted. When I was sitting in the train, a young black mother boarded with her three beautiful children. Their hair was spotlessly clean. Both mother and her three children looked happy, but I asked myself why these beautiful children had such pudding faces. I discovered the answer quickly, as I could see what the mother was dishing out to these children: coloured sweeties, chocolates and fizzy drinks. They were sitting on the other side of the corridor and, as there was a place next to me, the eldest girl (who was about seven or eight) came to sit beside me. Although there was no conversation, the girl looked at me as I was starting on my usual banana, and I asked her if she would like to share it with me. Wisely, the girl glanced at her mother for permission first, who nodded that she could, and we both had half a banana. As the train passed Tottenham Hale, it suddenly stopped quite abruptly. The little girl took my hand in shock and looked at me, and I calmed her down. When the train started to go again, she was tired and quite happily put her little head against my shoulder and slept all the way to Stansted. The mother, busy with the other two children, never spoke a word. I wish I'd had an opportunity to talk to her about her children's diet, but unfortunately I couldn't. When the train stopped in Stansted, I wakened the little girl quietly. She looked up to me with those beautiful dark eyes and said, 'Thank you for being my daddy.' That really was very touching and it made me think about how wonderful it is to have responsibility for children.

My mind went to my own ten grandchildren, and I thought of today's society in which these children grow up, the care that we give them and the love that they need to cope with life in the 21st century. Of course, to nature or to nurture is a very personal choice. I have seen parents in my day who made a lot of fuss if their child had a little fall or suffered a tiny scratch, and I have watched these children growing up into little hypochondriacs. I have also seen parents who just pooh-poohed every scratch, graze or fall, and who perhaps made their children too hard.

There is a balance in everything, but nature very often takes its own course. If we have a small scratch, it is best to allow nature to heal it. When children grow up with this attitude, they will be influenced by how we approach their problems and will let nature take over. I have lived in countries where babies were born in the most bizarre circumstances. These children grow up to be very independent, learning to cope with whatever life may bring.

My own children were all born at home and it was a wonderful experience to see from the very beginning what happened after they came to earth. I studied their little heartbeats, their hearing and swallowing, and watched their first reactions to life, which I always think is such a great wonder. Once the babies were fed, it was very interesting see how they developed, both physically and personally. My youngest grandchild, who has just been born, came to earth fully aware of all that was happening and, after a little while, developed the sort of personality that I saw in my own mother. On observation, there was the same twinkle that my mother used to have. It is a wonderful thing to think that those children and grandchildren bear the characteristics of parents and grandparents as they grow up, and how their personalities are formed. Some are there immediately and some develop slowly. Some babies have to fight, as one of my grandchildren did when she was born. It was her will and resistance that kept her alive, for she weighed just 1lb 8oz. It was clear that physical contact for this tiny baby did everything to help her fight for the life that she had been given. The feeling of being confident, safe and warm was very important and to let nature take its course is one of the most wonderful things.

It is also terribly important that, as a mother, you take care of yourself. Problems might arise such as jealousy or post-natal depression, and possibly even a feeling of anti-climax, as I discuss in my book *Pregnancy and Childbirth*. Do be open about it, talk about it and get advice about what remedies it may be necessary to take in order to meet the needs of your body. I have often seen that one simple mineral may be lacking at this time, zinc, and it may be necessary to take a zinc supplement.

Babies have a terrific sense of smell. This is a gift from nature and it is very important that small babies, once they have come to earth, smell, 'This is my mummy.' They are also very tuned into sounds and the sound of Mummy's or Daddy's voice is very important. Believe it or not, babies can also see. For the first two months, babies can see things most clearly when they are about eight inches from the bridge of the nose. Things go a bit out of focus when they are a bit further away. The most amazing thing is that a baby will always see the waving of a tree and will be very interested, when you walk under one, to see the leaves of the tree moving. It is very important to get the baby tuned into nature.

Sleep is one of the most important things for babies. Babies know how much sleep they needs. Once they have had enough, they will waken and will not go back to sleep, no matter what one does to try and make this happen. Often it is a question of getting the baby used to a routine. If natural sleep does not happen quickly enough, it is good, in order to make sure babies get a little rest, to give them ten drops of V*alerian hop*s before they go to bed.

Nature will tell babies when they are hungry. Regular feeding times are important, as this helps them understand routine. Follow your own feelings about this, as you will come to know your own child better than anybody else. The baby loves his or her mother the best of all. It is a good idea to naturally help babies when feeding by giving them little strokes and thinking loving thoughts – vibrations are very important. There are plenty of books available from the Health Service and the Education Board that will educate you on how to feed your baby. The material you use is important, and will help you to monitor your baby's development.

Babies' bowels must be looked after and there is nothing more important than allowing them to use their bowels naturally. It is important to learn and read a lot about toilet training. If there is a problem in the form of constipation, there are natural remedies to help. I often see with breast-fed babies who have soft stools (they are basically never hard) that if there is slight constipation, laxatives are certainly not the answer. Bottle-fed babies often become constipated. Their stools are usually harder and smellier than those of breast-fed babies. Natural foods like prune juice and sometimes a little yoghurt can remedy this. When there is such a problem, you can also give the baby natural remedies to help. For example, if the baby develops a sore bottom you may use a soft herbal ointment like *Ung Em*, made by the herbalists Abbots of Leigh especially for this problem, as well as nappy rash. It is a very safe remedy for the relief of discomfort.

Having practised homoeopathy for almost 45 years, I have seen how very beneficial homoeopathy is in looking after children. One of the finest ways to help children is to learn to understand the four principles of homoeopathy, one of them being to see what kind of character the baby develops and then use similar remedies. In other words, 'like cures like'. We often see that if the baby is a certain type, for instance *Belladonna, Gelsemium* or *Pulsatilla*, the very low potency remedies will quickly be effective. One of the other principles of homoeopathy is to look at the cause of a problem. It is often the case that children are bombarded with certain medicines to cure the symptoms of childhood illnesses and then run into more health problems at a later stage. Let nature take its course and when there is chickenpox, mumps or measles, always make sure that they get it well out of their systems as quickly as possible. Today, after all these years in practice, I have seen so many patients who have been the victims of not being properly treated when they had childhood illnesses. I am convinced that some of the degenerative diseases patients suffer from, such as multiple sclerosis, have their roots in the wrong treatment of childhood illnesses. Many men are sterile as a result of mumps. It is therefore very important that these particular problems are treated properly at the time. I have seen many people who couldn't have children at first, but who, after using homoeopathy to treat the miasmas which were left in their systems from former inflammation, viruses or infections, have become happy fathers and mothers.

Nature will always heal and, as my grandmother always said, 'Give me a flu and I will treat every illness.' In other words, a temperature that produces a sweat might sometimes be very necessary. Although medical care is important, please remember that if there is an imbalance in the body it should be removed from the system before it becomes a problem. Homoeopathy is certainly not a piece of chocolate, as one professor said. It deals with the causes of problems and it is very necessary in treating the child. When the child grows up nature will take its course, but nature needs to be given a chance. We so often want to feel well quickly, and we want the same thing for our children, but please help them with minor health problems by looking after them naturally.

The very first thing I look for when a baby is born is how well he or she breathes. Breathing is very important, and while the paediatrician thought one of my grandchildren would die, I knew she would live because she arrived breathing from the tummy. The breath of life was quite clearly seen in this baby and she has now developed into a lovely child who has no problems at all. When the baby grows up and its character starts to form, it is often the case that a relaxed child breathes in the tummy, whilst a very nervous or hyperactive child breathes above the tummy or in the chest, which is also the case with asthmatic children. It is very important to teach that child Hara breathing: inhaling through the nose, filling up the tummy with air and exhaling through the mouth in a nice, rhythmic manner. This sort of education is very important for the child.

It is a tremendous gift of God to have a child entrusted to you and that child, who depends on you completely and loves you, needs to know how much you love him or her. This determines a lot in later life, such as how much the child will be attached to you and how much influence you will then have when you want to protect the child when they meets situations that, as a parent, you can see are not good for him or her. Often, the best thing is to follow the voice of nature.

When I got married, I said to my wife, as she was in education and knew a lot more about children than I did, that I would back her decisions even if I did not always agree with them. Later, when we had children, we usually discussed both ways of thinking as to what was best for the child. Our task in making these decisions was even greater as we were both busy with our work and our children had to depend a lot on nannies. Although, thankfully, we had very good nannies, there were of course things we had to discuss in order to bring the children up in the best possible way, and secure their futures. We both knew that our children were confident that they were always very greatly cared for – something that I personally missed out on a lot in my own life.

As I mentioned in the Introduction, I asked Maria and Marcus to work on this book with me, to tell me their views on bringing up children. This is a very personal matter, but it is quite important for the child's health and well-being that some experienced advice is given. I once heard a couple asking an older, childless person how they should bring up their children. The older man asked what age the child was, and when he was told the child was five, he then said, 'You are too late. You should have made up your minds when your child was born on how to bring it up.' This sort of advice, however, requires the experience of people who have had children and who know the kinds of problems that can arise. For all of us, each day brings new experiences, especially for a child who is only just awakening to life. Each day new things happen for a child. He or she will have many questions about these new experiences, which need honest answers from a parent.

TWO

Baby – Small or Big

Quite some time ago my youngest daughter informed me she was pregnant. I was very happy. After eight weeks, her husband, although working in medicine, told me that on the scan the baby looked like 'a little cashew nut'. He showed me the scan – everything looked marvellous, and I thought then what a great wonder it all was. Sixteen weeks later, he showed me another scan and I saw that the baby had grown very well. I told him that all these scans were very, very nice to see, but I wasn't over-keen on them for pregnant women, and thought that my daughter shouldn't have too many scans. The pregnancy went very well and today when I look at their lovely boy and see how lively he is, I think of that little cashew nut and it makes me very happy.

A while later, my third daughter told me that she was pregnant. However, I was very worried about her health as she was not really made for having babies. Her pregnancy didn't go too well and she'd had a few miscarriages in the past. At one point, unfortunately, some mistakes were made during her pregnancy and I was very worried at times. Things progressed all right, though, but towards the sixth month her doctor, with whom she was quite friendly, became very worried and phoned to tell me that because of my daughter's high blood pressure and other complications, the baby had to be delivered straight away. She advised my daughter to go to the hospital to have the baby. When my granddaughter was born she was no more than about the weight of a packet of sugar – 1lb 8oz.

There wasn't much hope that she would live, but when I saw the baby, I assured my daughter and son-in-law, as well as some of the doctors, that I felt she would be all right. Her breathing was absolutely wonderful. There is a lot going for a baby who is born with the breath of life. This baby had wonderful rhythmic breathing and terrific willpower to live and, although she was on all kinds of monitors and leads, she tried very hard to get rid of them and wanted very much to be alive. She certainly was a very small baby, but her spirit was stronger than anything else and I felt so happy to see that this child was so lively. However, although she was given the breath of life, after a little while her tummy started to swell, and kept swelling like a big balloon until the doctor in charge felt that she had to be operated on as, of course, things were not in order. Her digestive system, being very immature, was not working the way it should and she had never passed a motion. We were, of course, all panicking when my son-in-law phoned to tell me that an operation had to be carried out. I worried my head off about what to do until suddenly, in the middle of the night, I got the answer. I phoned my son-in-law and told him that I couldn't help in the way I had thought of because I was only the grandfather but he, as the father, should go up to the hospital immediately and do exactly what I said. I thought of the healing methods that I had learned many years ago in India. I told him to ignore the nurses, wash his hands very well, go to her incubator, put his left hand on her tummy (right under the naval) and place his right hand over it, and hold it there with the breathing of his little child. He phoned me some time later to say that he had done this, but had got a terrible pain in his left arm and could no longer keep his hands on his child's tummy, so he had to remove them. Then the miracle happened – she passed her first motion. This baby, who was so small, developed well, although in six weeks, despite more than doubling her weight, she had only gone up to 5lb. Luckily, she was then allowed to go home and I can only say it is very special to have her, as well developed as she is now at the age of six, a really nice, intelligent young lady who knows exactly what she wants. So, things worked out all right.

There are often worries when babies are born prematurely, or when their births have to be induced because they are too late, at which time good care is necessary. Luckily, baby care in our country is absolutely excellent. I was so pleased with the care that my little grandchild received that I organised a very successful fundraising evening to help buy more of the machinery which was needed in that hospital.

One has to be careful, however, of what one is doing, despite the good standards of baby care in hospitals, and it is very important to look at what kind of food the baby is getting and at what one can do oneself to help, especially with digestive problems. The power of touch can indeed work miracles on newborn babies, and in my book *Body Energy* I have written a lot about this.

When a child is born either too big or too small, or develops at a different rate to that of other children, extra care is necessary. The child's health depends on what kind of food we choose, which to me seems logical. There is a lot of advice available on how to monitor the development of a child. It is very important as children grow up to realise that if they are too small, they will need reassurance. This was the greatest problem in my own young life; because I was very small in height, I developed an inferiority complex at a fairly early age, especially during World War Two when I was only about seven years old. Not only was I very small but I was also very thin. When the war was over, I was about eight years of age and just two and a half stones in weight. It was very difficult for me to battle my way through this because I was called all kinds of names. I was told that because I was small, I could not do this and I could not do that. If it hadn't been for the loving care of my family, from my mother especially, I would have been left with an inferiority complex as a result. So, it is important that we observe our children's development carefully and give the care that is needed, taking guidance from those with experience, especially in the first six months of parenthood. When babies are notably big or small, the first weeks after the baby's birth bring big changes. As there is no such thing as an absolutely perfect mother, it is very necessary to get the help of professionals.

When coping with wind, flatulence and especially colic, often caused by babies taking in too much air when feeding, it is often necessary to give them massages. This is especially important for babies that are very small. Gently rub the tummy and the back. This will result in better digestion, and the baby may even grow a little bit better because of this. Alternatively, you can simply slice an onion and dip it in very hot water a few times. Let the water become lukewarm, then give the baby a teaspoonful. If that doesn't help, it will do no harm to give him or her some fennel water or even two drops of *Septronium*, which can often be of the greatest help. Make sure that mealtimes are always happy and follow professional guidelines to help the baby. I would, however, advise caution if allergic reactions appear. There is more about this later, in Chapter Eight.

Don't forget that the first six months, whether babies are big or small, are very important. Although in some cases development might be faster than others, it is very important that one observes carefully and notices when the baby can support his or her own head, begins to look properly at human faces, starts to smile or looks at certain objects to play with. It is also important to monitor all the movements the baby makes. If the baby has been born with a little force, either by forceps or other methods, after six weeks it might be a good idea to consult a reputable cranial osteopath, who will look carefully at the skull for any possible damage that may have been done. I recently had a case of a very big baby whose mother was extremely emotional during pregnancy because she had lost her husband and had many worries. This baby was born with the help of forceps, and afterwards suffered epileptic fits every five minutes. None of the drugs that were administered were of any help and when she finally brought this baby to me, I had to adjust the skull slightly. Luckily, no drugs were necessary after that and the epileptic fits stopped.

It is very important that if a baby has problems with movement, or misalignments in its body, a qualified osteopath is consulted, as they can often be of great help. Defects should be attended to. One should not always take the attitude that everything will turn out all right in the end, as some form of treatment or adjustment may be necessary. I have often said to students that if Isaac Newton had known when he discovered the laws of gravity that he would contribute so much to medicine today he would have been happy, for we know now that the centre of gravity is very important. A baby who has the wrong centre of gravity needs to be readjusted. Just as when a wheel in a watch is out of balance and the watch stops, or a ship loaded too much on one side keels over, so the baby, later in life, will have problems if the misalignment is not attended to. Extra help is available from qualified practitioners if it is needed. But give it some time at first, especially as the first few days after the baby is born are so special; nature will very often make the necessary adjustments. The first few weeks are also important. Then all kinds of problems can arise, such as clicking hips, club feet, cleft palates or hernias. There is a lot of help at hand for problems like these.

Of course, the baby's weight is of very great importance. Watch closely to see if your baby is happy and content, and is gaining weight normally. In the first few weeks, most babies gain about six to eight ounces (170–227g) a week, but this usually slows down to about four or five ounces a week after the first three months. The average baby's birth weight usually doubles by the age of five months, and trebles by the time the baby is one year old. Do remember that a baby is an individual; one is not the same as another and it is best that each be monitored and assessed individually. As I will write later on the nature or nurture issue, it is very important that a newborn child can adapt to a different environment if it is necessary. During the nine months from conception to birth, growth is of the same absolute magnitude as in further years.

Ten Things I Learned About Life from Giving Birth
By Theresa Pitman, Oakville, Ontario

1. Sometimes things hurt – emotionally as well as physically – and the best you can do is try to relax and know it will stop hurting eventually. Trying to stop the hurt with drugs or pretending it isn't happening doesn't work very well and can make you miss out on important parts of life. Pain comes, but it goes away again.
2. Being in control isn't always possible or even desirable. Sometimes you have to just let things happen.
3. Listen to your body, it has the wisdom of generations and will guide you well if you let it. Your body can teach you about eating and exercising and making love and just living as well as giving birth and breast-feeding.
4. Life is often messy and unpredictable; we are closer to nature than we think we are, and at no time is that clearer than when we are giving birth.

5. Keep people who support you and care for you around as much as possible and avoid people who only drain energy from you and make you feel worse. In labour, the right person can make you feel courageous and capable and the wrong person can make you feel inadequate and suffering. It's exactly the same in the rest of our lives.

6. You are stronger than you think you are. You can cope with things you never thought you could cope with.

7. Life is full of small, everyday miracles. A baby is one of them – so is a sunrise, a smile, or the existence of life.

8. Every day the world is being born again, and we can begin again. Every baby is a new beginning, but every moment can be for all of us.

9. Our capacity to love is many times larger than we think. Having four children to love does not mean we love each of them one-quarter as much as we would one child. Love expands.

10. Those who really love us will love us for ourselves, without any need for pretending. My babies loved my singing, even though nobody else ever did and as they've grown they've come to love my odd sense of humour and my less-than-spotless housekeeping. If we can be ourselves as we give birth, and have that self accepted, we can be ourselves in the rest of our lives.

THREE

Mother and Child Relationship

The first thing that a baby needs is air, the second thing a baby needs is food and the third thing a baby needs is love. If the last of these is not there, the baby will starve. It is very important that during pregnancy the mother experiences love for her baby, and when the baby is born, it is important that he or she feels loved straight away. We see this not only in humans, but also in the animal kingdom. Love is one of the most important requirements for a healthy, happy baby.

Whilst I am writing this book, thinking of my children, I feel very guilty. The reason that I feel guilty is because I have worked so hard in my life, wanting to secure a future for my children, that I have very much neglected the loving relationship that was so necessary when they were growing up. Our children were looked after by nannies as both my wife and I were very busy, working hard to secure a future for the children so that they could study and could get on in life. Then I was so concerned with this that I forgot I should be spending a lot more time with my children, and I am very pleased to see that they haven't made the same mistake with their own children. It is a wonderful thing when I see my children and grandchildren together, looking at each one of them while they are growing up, seeing how they have established themselves and how they have learned to cope with what life brings them. I have also seen that the guilt I carry with me in not always giving the time I should has not rubbed off on my children. They have wonderful relationships with their own children. I often look back and think how precious those moments really were, when I took them cycling or walking, or even just spent some quality time with them. As I get older, these precious moments are often of the greatest comfort to me in times when I feel a bit low.

My own childhood was a very difficult one, as I grew up in a world full of anger, war and murder. My comfort was my mother, as my father and my brother were taken away by the Nazis. In that particular period, my mother was very busy with underground work, hiding people who were hunted by the Nazis but not forgetting to give me the time that I needed and to comfort me. At that particular time of great need, a special relationship developed between my mother and myself. I could go to her with the worries I had and my terrible fear that the Germans would shoot her because of the work she was doing. The bond was there and I would always ask my mother for advice when I grew older. A relationship developed which I treasured till the day she died. Her spirit, however, is still with me every day. How very important the mother and child relationship is, and what a responsibility.

My brother, a real sportsman, was ten times better a father than I. He had a very close relationship with his children, as did his wife. However, when he died, his children were totally devastated and I could see the mistake that my brother and I had both made in not sensibly bringing up the children to cope when the loss of one of their parents came. We have to develop a strong relationship with our children so that they can cope with loss and sadness in life. It is very important in the mother and child relationship to be sensible and have an understanding of the real needs of a child.

I once read a book written by Helen Bethune called *Positive Parent Power*. It gives a seven-part programme on how to deal with the problems that children will have. She says in the introduction of the book something that is very true: 'It is the parents' job to look at how parents could do more or should do more and, whatever the circumstances, parents are supposed to know what to do for the best and what is in the best interest of their child.' There is so much confusion over this particular issue. I liked the seven points she makes about the different types of power: biological power; legitimate power; diagnostic power; coercive power; reward power; moral power; and personal power. Regarding those points, she makes very interesting remarks about the significance of the blood type of the child, and the help and protection we give to it. She also remarks that instinct is not love, although the two are frequently confused. But although love can be selfish, it is not possessive and loving parents will do everything possible for the good of their child.

My mother, a very wise woman, always said that children are only lent to us for a short while and we have to learn that although the mother and child relationship is very important one day we will have to leave our children alone. We have to bring them up to the best of our ability so that they can cope with life on their own, setting them a good example ourselves. Not long before my mother died, she called me and said: 'You have wonderful children and I know that you hang on to them, but I will give you some advice. Children will want their own space, they will want to make their own decisions and you have to leave them alone no matter what direction they choose to take. If they take the dining-room chairs and stick them to the ceiling, keep your mouth shut. It is none of your business any more. It is their life and if they want to cope with it that way, do not interfere.'

Over the years, being a grandfather, I have often learned the hard way to keep my mouth shut. This can be for the better, as one can very easily damage one's relationship with children by attempting to have what might be a slightly selfish influence on them. It is the responsibility of parents to adapt in order to prevent our children from feeling that they are being manipulated by us, or influenced by the way we think. We should treat them with respect and as parents we must earn respect, because it is not a right.

The kind of image we present is very important, and so is the kind of guidance we give to our children. Our responsibilities as parents have changed in the 21st century. One has to be realistic. Using our influence is a very great thing, but we have to ask ourselves how our children see us and what our advice can offer them. We should not only give our children shelter and protection, food and sustenance, but also a sense of order. They need to know that we love them very much and that we will only give them sensible rules. We have to be as positive as we possibly can, and give them the realisation that they will get out of life what they are willing to put into it. Being an adequate parent means giving children the understanding that they need to have a relationship, and not letting them starve of air or food, or of the love that is necessary to bind them to us.

One of the greatest problems nowadays in this permissive world is teaching the child moral power, the everyday morality that is learnt from example. We must not use excuses or white lies, and have to teach children honesty, respect and discipline – not an easy thing to do in a world where there are so many adverse influences. It is fascinating when we look at children, however, how much innate moral sensibility they have when they are born, principles that their parents and grandparents also have. It is quite interesting to see how young children have an integral understanding of what is right and wrong. They do not learn this only from their parents' example, but have an in-built moral core that manifests itself in a feeling of responsibility even in very young children. Nowadays honesty is a very, very difficult thing to maintain, and unless we teach our children that value, with so many dishonest influences in the world the child will be under tremendous attack. This means that, as parents, we have to be honest in everything. I have often seen that when either myself or other parents go wrong in not giving the full truth, the child picks this up very quickly and will then use the same sort of excuses, based on dishonesty, and this can go from bad to worse.

In my work in British prisons, I have often seen how criminality was born into offenders as young children because their parents were either dishonest or sowing seeds of doubt and fear in these little hearts. As they grew up, this led some of them to become life-sentence prisoners. For these people, I feel sorry because they are not wholly guilty of the problems they have caused. These are often due to their upbringing at home, which was the basis of the criminal lives that they lead. We must not forget that children always look up to their parents as being on the highest pedestal and what the parents do they take as gospel truth, believing that they can do it as well. If we have a clear conscience and are responsible, this will always work positively in our children and grandchildren. The greatest seeds of responsibility can unconsciously lie in them after they are born.

Enjoy your lives with your babies, get to know all about the little things that they do and work with your own feelings and theirs to bring about a harmonious relationship that will form the basis of your future together. Children have needs and we all meet them in different ways. Parental love, especially a mother's, is of immeasurable importance from birth. A mother and child's relationship consists basically of love and security. In the 21st century, children are very vulnerable and at risk. Willpower and determination are necessary and in my practice I have often seen problems of lack of confidence when there was trouble at home (either emotional, or problems between father and mother). The important thing is that whatever the circumstances, the child has a feeling of security and knows how to cope with little difficulties, whether mental, physical or emotional. Mental stimulation is necessary and when the child is bored or not cooperating, it is then that the mother and child relationship is terribly important.

Working mothers have a big responsibility. The child, who has a right to be well looked after, must have childcare provided by capable people. Always look either to a family member, such as a grandmother, or another very caring person to look after the child. Although my wife and I were very busy, we spent a lot of time and money finding the best nannies that we could, and felt safe in the knowledge that our children were in good care. Later on in life this will pay dividends. Children need to have the confidence and the security to know that, wherever they are, they are well cared for and looked after in the best way possible. Mothers should have the right to refuse shift work if the children are at home. Children are usually safe and secure at school, and they should find the same security back at home, with their mother there. Although male colleagues might be angry about this, it is of the greatest importance for family life that children are well looked after. It might be a bit inconvenient for companies, but nevertheless it is important that the mother is free at times when the children are at home.

The other day I saw a very well-known actress in my clinic in London. I asked her how she was getting on and her answer was quite simple: 'In the first place, I am a mother and my first priority is my children to whom, in my busy life, I give all my attention. In the second place, I am an actress and I believe I am a good actress, as I am often asked for.' She is indeed – she is brilliant – but her priorities are right and because of that she does both jobs very well, giving her husband and children first place. This positive attitude makes the combination of working and being a mother work very well. When one is positive, one very often gets positive results. Imagine that all will work out as it should and with that in mind, it mostly will. The failures that I have seen are caused by negativity. Positive will always win over negative, not the other way around, as I often say, and balance is very important.

A young mother who came to see me the other day had several problems, and her children told me that she would not know what to do without her grandmother, who was in her 90s. She said her grandmother was not only a grandmother, but often a mother to whom she could go with a lot of her problems. At her age, she still wanted to be both a mother and a grandmother and because of that she was greatly loved.

FOUR

Breast or Bottle?

This first major decision facing new parents often causes great anxiety and controversy. For such a personal issue, it can seem that advice abounds from everyone – experts and in-laws alike – leaving the first-time mother in particular confused and worried. Although health experts justifiably argue that 'breast is best', there are other issues to take into consideration.

Breast-feeding can often be seen as the easy option due to the lack of the time-consuming task of heating and sterilising bottles. In reality, breast-feeding often comes with problems (although, on the whole, these can be overcome). Often painful initially, breast-feeding has left many mothers in tears, especially in the middle of the night, when it can be lonely and frustrating as the tiny baby cries out for food. Although these times can be hard, the good news is that once breast-feeding has become established, most women agree, with hindsight, that it was a worthwhile and fulfilling experience.

It's common knowledge that breast milk is superior to formula milk – it is, after all, what nature provided to feed our children, but there are certain circumstances when formula milk should be considered. A stressed mother, for instance, will find it hard to provide the amount and quality of milk her little baby may need; twins can prove demanding on the milk supply, leaving mothers drained of energy, and babies in intensive care need to have their food quality and consumption monitored very closely.

The demands of our modern lifestyle are dramatically different from those of a century ago, and although domestic chores are easier due to modern equipment, this has led to an increased availability of time which most people fill with day-to-day rushing around. Added to this, the pressures of society to get 'back to normal', get back to work and integrate our offspring into our busy lives often lead to problems, especially when it comes to breast-feeding. The 'feed on demand' regime of breast-feeding can simply make it too difficult to incorporate into a hectic lifestyle, with the quality of milk suffering; often it is simply easier for a bottle-feeding routine to be established.

In the Western world, breast-feeding in public is still not wholly acceptable to many, leaving the majority of women little choice but to retreat to the toilets to feed their little one. One answer to overcoming this could lie in expressing the milk. This, however, often brings its own problems. It is time-consuming, and it does alter the natural milk flow, confusing the body as to the amount of milk needed. Often, as a result, too much or too little milk is produced which, in turn, has an effect on the amount of milk the baby receives when returning to breast-feeding. The balance may be upset and the body compensates for this. If the breasts produce too much milk, they may become engorged. This is not only painful but, more importantly, if left untreated, can lead to mastitis, an inflammatory condition of the breast. If too little milk is produced, the baby will demand his or her feeds more often which can, in the longer term, cause the breasts to produce more milk – which can then cause the complications outlined above. For mothers returning to work, expressing the milk does have a major benefit, however, as it allows the baby to be nourished in her absence.

When choosing between bottle and breast, it is worth keeping the basic principles of nature in mind. Nature has provided our body – if we calm down, relax and give the body the chance it deserves – with food that changes according to our exact needs. The amount of protein, fat, sugar (lactose) and other components in breast milk alters to suit the baby's needs at any given time.

Milk is the ideal food for any baby, but there are many different kinds of milk and each kind has a different composition. Horses' milk contains exactly what the foal needs, goats' milk is good for the little kid, etc. Every mammal on earth needs exclusively the milk from its own kind. A calf grows much faster than a human baby and, because of this, cows' milk contains much more calcium, phosphorus and protein than human milk. Mothers' milk contains almost twice as much sugar (lactose) than cows' milk, and the quality of the milk sugar is totally different.

This lactose is instrumental in developing the bacterial flora – the much-needed bacteria in the baby's intestines, which protect the baby from illness. Also, lactose is indispensable for the body's own production of myelin, a kind of fat that surrounds the nerve fibres. When these nerves are not protected enough, serious diseases of the nervous system like, for example, multiple sclerosis, can develop. Scientists in New Zealand have researched these connections in great detail. Also leukaemia and some kinds of cancer seem to tie up with the consumption of cows' milk.

The fat content of mothers' milk and cows' milk is almost the same, but there is a great difference in quality. Mothers' milk contains more specific fatty acids, which are very important for the development of the nerves and the brain of the baby. The fat and other substances found in cows' milk hardly have any value for the human body, as their quality is completely different. A baby fed only on cows' milk grows faster and often gains more weight than a baby who drinks mothers' milk. However, breast-fed babies usually have no digestive problems, their defence system functions better, and their mental and spiritual development is superior.

In the stomach of a newborn baby there are completely different enzymes from those found in the stomach of small children and grown-ups. As the baby grows, the composition of the gastric juices gradually changes. After this, the digestive system is prepared to handle a different kind of food.

Another benefit of breast-feeding is that the body can also produce the exact amount of milk to meet the baby's demands. When the baby sucks the breast, an area in the brain (the hypothalamus) is stimulated, which sends signals to the pituitary gland at the base of the brain. A hormone, *oxytocin*, is then released into the bloodstream. *Oxytocin* flows into the breast and causes cells around the milk glands to contract. Some milk – the foremilk – collects in the ducts behind the nipple. This thirst-quenching milk is low in calories and high in protein and will keep the baby satisfied until *oxytocin* causes the let-down reflex (the small muscles around the area where the milk is stored in the breasts contract and the milk is squeezed out). This releases the more calorific, satisfying hind milk. *Prolactin*, another hormone, stimulates the brain which sends a signal to the breast to make more milk.

This amazing biological system is not the only reason to choose breast-feeding. It is a fact that breast-fed babies are less likely to develop allergies. They are also less prone to illness, due to the protective antibodies they receive from their mother, and let's not forget that breast milk is easily digested and comes at the right temperature, so stomach problems, such as constipation, are not as common. Breast-fed babies are also less prone to nappy rash because their stools do not contain the bacteria which generally causes ammonia dermatitis, a condition that comes about when urine mixes with bacteria in the stools, creating ammonia, which leads to irritation.

Breast-feeding also encourages the womb to contract and the excess fat accumulated during pregnancy is used up, so the pre-pregnancy figure returns more quickly. Perhaps the most important justification for breast-feeding is that it enhances bonding. Once the umbilical cord has been cut, the baby and mother are separated and it is up to the mother to stay connected with her young one at this tender age. Breast-feeding offers a unique opportunity for both mother and baby to come close, and this is further enhanced if some quiet time is taken together away from the hustle and bustle of life.

If the decision between bottle and breast-feeding is still a concern, it is worth remembering that it is easier to start breast-feeding and then stop than to start bottle-feeding and then try to switch to the breast. Bear in mind that during the first few days after birth the breast produces a special sort of milk, colostrum, which is rich in protein. Most importantly, it contains vital antibodies which are beneficial to help resist disease. It also acts as a laxative, helping babies to pass their first stool.

Many women who are unsure about which form of feeding they are going to choose are swayed by their own mothers. This is often entirely dependent on what the accepted norm was at that time. In the '60s and '70s bottle-feeding was the recommended feeding plan.

Now, health professionals try to push for breast-feeding, but often hospital staff find bottle-feeding much easier on their workloads and timetables. It is easy to imagine that if you were the only woman on the ward breast-feeding, the tangible pressure from the other women, as the baby cries for milk, would be enough to sway a new mum into bottle-feeding.

The majority of Western women need to be taught how to breast-feed their baby. It is thought that this is due to us not seeing women feeding their babies in public. For successful breast-feeding, you need to be relaxed and comfortable before you start feeding (hunching your shoulders can also reduce milk flow). Gentle breathing exercises are essential for successful breast-feeding. The simplest method is to place your hands on your stomach and slowly take a breath in through your nose, deep enough to make your hands rise, and then slowly control the breath out through the mouth. Repeat this as many times as you need to, until you feel your breathing become slow, steady and controlled.

Support is essential in the early days of breast-feeding. Milk flow is affected by emotions and with the highs and lows in the first few weeks after the birth, the let-down reflex can be altered so that milk flow slows or stops altogether. Often, it is at this point that women either 'give up' or are told they are not producing enough milk. To overcome this, try taking some flax oil. It has been shown that this will not only enhance the quality and quantity of the milk, but also helps the development of the baby's brain and nervous system.

Whatever method you choose to feed your baby, the most important consideration is to enjoy your newborn to the full. Any mother will inform you that these early years 'fly by' and this is not time that can be regained or 'made up' at some later date. If, however, you are finding breast-feeding tough and painful, and it is impeding your mental outlook towards yourself and the baby, you may have good reason to start bottle-feeding. On the other hand, if you persevere, it could be the best decision you make and you will always remember that special time with your young baby.

Table 1: Beating Breast-feeding Blues

Engorged Breasts	Heavy, uncomfortable breasts are common, especially between two to four days after the birth. It is due to milk rather than the initial colostrum.
What To Do	Alternate hot and cold flannels on the breasts. Place a cabbage leaf in your bra to take the heat and inflammation out of the breast. Massage the breasts gently from the outside in towards the nipple with almond oil.
Sore/Cracked Nipples	This is usually due to the baby not being 'latched on' properly. Poor positioning of yourself and the baby can pull on the nipple and can cause this very painful condition.
What To Do	Ensure the baby latches on properly each time. After feeding, break the suction by placing your little finger inside the mouth and opening the baby's jaw slightly. Check that your posture is relaxed and your baby is positioned so that he or she is not pulling at your breast. Try applying calendula or chamomile cream to the sore or cracked areas.
Mastitis	This is a serious complaint of breast-feeding. It is usually the result of a lump that does not drain completely when feeding, leading to infection. Symptoms include fever, dizziness, high temperatures and redness in the breast.
What To Do	Check with your health visitor or midwife, because if left untreated, it can develop into an abscess. Place a warm flannel against the tender area to encourage milk flow. Massage the area with warm oil. After massaging, place a cabbage leaf over the area.

	Repeat the process regularly.
	Echinacea can help the infection as it acts as a natural antibiotic.
	If it does not clear in 48 hours, it may be necessary to take antibiotics to prevent a breast abscess from developing.
Low Milk Flow	This can be caused by anxiety, and sometimes the baby may not be latched on properly and if this is the case the breasts will not make more milk.
What To Do	Practice relaxation techniques before feeding. At the least, have a few quiet moments.
	Check your and your baby's positioning to ensure that he or she is latched on properly.
	Try drinking fennel tea to stimulate milk flow.
	Supplement your diet with flax seed capsules, which enhance the quality of the milk and stimulate milk flow.

DO WE NEED MILK?

Humans are the only creatures who still drink milk alien to their species, even when they are grown up, although their bodies are not equipped to digest it adequately. It is a known fact that adult milk drinkers can be found mostly in industrialised countries, where the percentage of caries of the teeth, hip-joint operations and diseases of the bones are the highest. Most surprisingly, many people in Africa and Asia, who never drink milk, have strong teeth and healthy bones.

Only a small percentage of the world's population drinks cows' milk. In antiquity and during the middle ages, cheese (especially goats' cheese) was eaten at times, but drinking milk was not a common habit, and goats' milk was usually only an *emergency solution* when feeding babies.

Later, cows' milk was used only sporadically until about 100 years ago. Then scientists discovered that milk contained many valuable substances. Since then, dairy products have grown into a billion-dollar industry, and milk is now recommended as one of the healthiest foods, even by many doctors.

Of course, raw, untreated cows' milk contains many vital substances. However, it seems that no one has realised that any food is only good for our health if our organism can metabolise it. Unfortunately, with cows' milk, this is often not the case. The problem with milk is that as soon as it comes into contact with oxygen, or has been heated or treated (pasteurised, etc.) in any way, its originally valuable ingredients change and become totally different substances. Many people have an allergic reaction to this milk, and are unable to metabolise the milk proteins or the milk sugar. The following section explains why this is so.

Certainly, while in most cases cows' milk will be suitable, I have found that with babies in general goats' milk is preferable and mostly prevents an allergic reaction.

THE CONNECTION BETWEEN CLIMATIC CONDITIONS AND MILK COMPATIBILITY

In southern countries, where the sun is nearly always shining and people eat more fish, the calcium supply for the population is practically guaranteed. In Asia and other countries where people do not drink milk, the calcium need is covered by soy products, seaweed, seafood, etc. Yet in northern countries, where the sun seldom shines and where, in former times, fruit and vegetables were only available during the short summer months, nature provided an emergency solution for the supply of calcium. Over many generations, people in those countries developed a gene which stimulated the production of lactose, which is needed for the digestion of milk. That is why, for instance, Scandinavians can digest milk and dairy products better than other Europeans.

Several years ago at the University of Heidelberg, it was confirmed that only 55 per cent of the inhabitants of Central Europe could digest cows' milk adequately. In southern countries, about 90 per cent of the population is unable to digest cows' milk completely.

Unfortunately, for financial reasons milk and dairy products are strongly promoted in these countries. This can have, as we have seen in African countries, for example, disastrous consequences. As the Third World countries still believe that the best things come from Western countries, many doctors there recommend cows' milk as the best food for babies and small children. Most of these doctors know very little about nutrition. Due to massive advertising campaigns and promotions, millions of children (e.g. in Spain and Italy) consume cows' milk almost daily, usually mixed with chocolate, for breakfast.

Chocolate, bread, cookies, crackers, etc., which contain *hidden milk*, do serious harm to consumers in these countries. As a result of wrong nutritional habits, many children become milk and/or sugar addicts; they become easily tired, ill or nervous, and nobody seems to know why.

THE DIFFERENT WAYS IN WHICH MILK IS PRODUCED

With every step of the treatment process milk loses more of its original value, and it is interesting to learn what one of Germany's greatest nutritional scientists, Prof. Kollath, had to say about this:

> Only raw milk is completely natural. This kind of milk will always be the most valuable for our health. All products made from raw milk, like skimmed milk, buttermilk, whey and, of course, butter and fresh cream, can be regarded as second best, although they are still very healthy and valuable. They can even be eaten by children and adults who otherwise have allergic reactions when eating dairy products. Butter and fresh cream contain mainly milk fat, which is easier to digest than milk protein or milk sugar.
>
> All types of milk which have been through a fermentation process, like sour milk, yoghurt, kefir, cottage cheese and quark – provided that they have been produced from raw milk – belong to the third category. They can still be recommended, but only when eaten in small quantities.
>
> In the fourth category, we find all heated products like, for example, pasteurised milk and dairy products made from pasteurised milk. When milk is heated, the protein molecules in the milk are damaged and this results in a loss of enzymes and vitamins. Protein in the human body is also damaged at a temperature of over 42ºC. As,

however, in some countries, the pasteurisation of milk is prescribed by law, one has to put up with these losses in value if one still wishes to drink milk.

Where milk is preserved by still higher, or by extremely high temperatures, as is the case with sterilised milk and all its by-products, all vital nutrients are destroyed. They belong to the fifth category.

The next is the sixth and last category of milk preservation. In this category, there is condensed or tinned milk, dried milk and milk powder for babies and small children. Because of the fact that manufacturers try to make their products resemble mothers' milk as much as possible, these powdered milk products receive an even more intensive treatment, thereby the loss in valuable and vital substances increases, and those few nutrients, which these products still contain, have undergone a complete change compared to the original product from which they were made. A mother who uses such milk products for her baby should realise that in this way her baby receives the least valuable food instead of the most valuable.

WHEN BABIES CANNOT DIGEST COWS' MILK

It often happens that babies do not have enough of the enzymes which are needed for the digestion of milk proteins. If indigestible milk residues cannot be eliminated in a normal way, the body will try to find another solution. Then these residues come out by way of the skin and the baby gets a skin rash, the so-called milk scab, infantile eczema, other skin problems and/or diarrhoea. If diarrhoea or skin problems are being suppressed with medicaments, this can eventually lead to the development of neurodermatitis, which is very difficult to cure.

The elimination of residues from the proteins of cows' milk puts a heavy stress on the baby's kidneys, which are still underdeveloped. Milk protein contains more than 25 different substances which, in combination with sugar or flour, can trigger allergic reactions. Among these are problems of behaviour, hyperactivity, nervousness, irritability and chronic fatigue, which are quite common today.

If these proteins irritate the urinary tract, they often cause bedwetting, even with older children. In the case of such a problem, one should try to leave milk and milk products out of the menu for at least a few weeks. Often we see that many such problems then disappear within a short time.

FIVE

Food, Mood, the Brain and Beyond

'We used to think our future was in the stars. Now we know it's in our genes.'
James Watson, Nobel laureate and co-discoverer of DNA

There is growing evidence that eating the correct diet may help prevent many disorders of the mind, such as epilepsy, schizophrenia, dementia and autism, but just how powerful is the influence of our diet compared to that of our genetic constitution? Viewed another way, maybe we should be considering the combined power of our genetic make-up and diet, since genes for certain disorders may only express themselves in special situations. For example, I think many psychiatrists agree that certain people have addictive personalities. In the presence of excess alcohol, the gene expresses itself and the person becomes an alcoholic. What is interesting is the fact that most reformed alcoholics often turn to another addiction, such as smoking or eating, to fill the gap in their lives. Those who win through and turn their backs on destructive addictions may find themselves following strict religious or work-based pursuits. Just as humans can become addicted to alcohol, so too can they become addicted to drugs. There is a growing body of evidence that suggests our genetics are at the root of these evils.

Studies of brains from alcoholics show that they have fewer dopamine receptors than non-alcoholics; maybe this was genetically determined. Genes have also been implicated in smokers. In one study of 283 smokers, over one-third had an unusual gene that was not present in non-smokers. This gene, named D2, was also found to be responsible for the low number of dopamine receptors discovered in the brains of alcoholics. Now we can start to see a strong genetic link developing between the two types of addiction. With one genetic defect, we can see two very different addictive behaviours, and potential lifestyle and health outcomes. Our addicts may be viewed as 'medicating' themselves, since both alcohol and smoking will elevate the dopamine levels (by blocking its re-uptake) and stimulate the pleasure centres deep within the brain. So too will certain foods, such as carbohydrates, since the release of another happy hormone, serotonin, occurs when we eat them.[1]

When it comes to a discussion on diet and health, the human brain must feel a bit left out. We are all aware that certain foods and vitamins feed our skin, a low animal fat diet is good for the heart, drinking plenty of water helps our kidneys, and our bones benefit from extra calcium, whilst the joints often feel better for an oiling up with a daily dose of cod liver oil. What about our brains? They have very special needs, but how many of us give this amazing structure a second thought?

Compared to the lightweight brain of our closest ancestor, the monkey, which weighs about 105 grams, the average human brain weighs in at a colossal 1,350 grams. From a developmental point of view, it is the first tissue to develop, at about 16 days after conception. Eating well is vital if you are trying to conceive, since you may not be aware that you are pregnant by the time your baby's brain has started to develop. Even though the brain forms only 2 per cent of our body weight, it uses around 50 per cent of the blood pumped from the heart, and consumes well over 20 per cent of the total body oxygen and glucose used each day. Such a high blood supply and fuel consumption shows how essential fresh supplies of food are for healthy brain function.

However, don't forget that the feeding of a healthy brain starts before birth! It has been said that the seeds of good adult health are sown before conception, during pregnancy and during infancy, the seeds of health being the specific nutrients contained in our daily diet. It has recently been discovered that certain oils (belonging to the fat family known as omega-3s) are essential for the normal development of the brain and nervous system during pregnancy. This reliance on the omega-3 fats continues for the first couple of years of life. One specific member of this fat family, known as docosahexaenoic acid (DHA) has the ability to stimulate the growth of the retina (the light-sensitive inner part of the eye) and the brain itself. DHA can, therefore, be considered to be a specific brain nutrient. Apart from the brain, DHA plays an important function in the correct functioning of the immune system.

The developing baby is reliant on his or her mother for an adequate DHA supply. Dietary intake accounts for the majority of DHA used by the baby and obtained through the placenta and, later on, in the breast milk. Many formula feeds are very low in DHA. In fact, the fat content of most formula feeds are based on commercially processed oils which contain high levels of potentially damaging fats known as 'trans-fatty acids'. It has been estimated that breast milk contains over 30 per cent more DHA than formula feeds: breast is always best!

Just take a trip around any supermarket and you will be confronted with an enormous and ever-growing variety of low-fat or fat-free food products. These foods are aimed at our obsession with low-fat diets promoted by the media. With our ever-growing knowledge about the importance of essential fatty acids, it is questionable if this new style of eating is the healthy option it is made out to be. However, this is not an invitation to throw caution to the wind and pig out on fatty foods. I would still advise moderation in animal (saturated) fats while increasing oily fish and foods high in monounsaturated fats – the good fats! The shift in modern eating habits is causing serious concern regarding the growing followers of the low-fat culture. This diet trend is causing a drop in the essential fatty acid intake in the general population. Most worrying is the potential adverse effects this may have on mothers-to-be and their babies' developing nervous systems.

Recently, the press announced the fact that the brains of pregnant women shrink over the course of their pregnancy. During the course of a study carried out at the Royal Postgraduate Medical School in which scientists were investigating the causes of pregnancy-related blood pressure problems, they stumbled across the unexpected finding that the brains of the women they were studying were shrinking. The investigating team discovered that the mothers were deficient in the essential fatty acids that were needed by the developing baby's brain and nervous system. Such was the demand that the stores contained in the mothers' brains were mobilised into the general circulation for delivery to the developing baby. The adult brain is a rich reserve pool of these special fats. Happily, however, the brains returned to normal after six to ten months, but the fact remains that the reserve pool was tapped into, demonstrating the absolute necessity for these fatty acids.

It is common knowledge that folic acid is essential for the healthy formation of the nervous system. Most pregnant mothers are now given tablets of 400 mcg folic acid to prevent spina bifida in their babies, but what about oil supplements? Deficiencies of the omega-3 family can lead to learning difficulties because of their importance in the development of the nervous system, but because learning and behavioural problems are only normally noticed some years after birth and are not life threatening, unlike spina bifida, they have not prompted much attention. There is a popular misconception that fats act as nothing more than storage systems for energy or as packing material. Only recently has it been acknowledged that fats have a very significant role in the metabolism and development of the body. There is a clear need for a greater understanding of the role of fatty acid metabolism in the maintenance of cell membrane health. There is evidence accumulating that any dietary programme aimed at helping an autistic child should involve a balance of both omega-3 and omega-6 fatty acids, rather than gross overloading of one form.[2] Evening primrose oil consists largely of gamma-linolenic acid (GLA), an omega-6 acid. There are other richer sources of GLA, such as borage (starflower) oil, but it is claimed that this is less well tolerated by most people than the oil from evening primrose. Fish oils, such as cod liver oil, have the added advantage of including supplementary vitamin A, which is likely to be in short supply in children with autism.

Flaxseed oil is a rich source of omega-3 acids. A daily dose of flaxseed oil will rebalance the situation. Taken at a dose of 1–2g a day, it will provide all the necessary fatty acids needed for health. Flaxseed oil is a richer supply of omega-3s than fish oil – almost twice as concentrated in fact. From the high content of GLA contained in flax oil, the body can make all the DHA it needs.

The adult brain is not a static structure. Our ideas about the brain have changed since the early days of neurology and its plasticity (the ability to change and adapt to different situations) has now been appreciated.

The chemical environment of the brain is all-important. Even minor nutritional deficiencies can have major implications for healthy brain function. It has been noted that symptoms of dementia can occur long before the levels of vitamin B12 and folic acid are shown to be low in blood tests. Vitamin B12 deficiency is not uncommon in Alzheimer's disease, further supporting the importance of a good nutritional balance. Unfortunately, by the time symptoms start to be noticed, supplementation may come too late. A long-term minor deficiency has been suggested to cause slow and irreversible changes in the nervous tissue, until it becomes unresponsive to corrective supplementation.

As with many nutritional substances, there is a good deal of interaction between the food chemicals that enter the brain. Vitamin C, for example, plays an essential part in the healthy action of another important brain food – the amino acid known as phenylalanine. Phenylalanine works to produce nerve-transmitting substances (called neurotransmitters) that regulate the electrical activity of the brain. Neurotransmitters are responsible for an elevated and positive mood, alertness and mental well-being; a lack causes many brain disorders, such as depression and schizophrenia.

As well as vitamin C, the mineral zinc has a part to play in mental health. It has been observed that many people suffering from irritability, nervousness and anxiety have higher than normal levels of copper circulating in their bodies. Copper and zinc have an interesting relationship in that a deficiency of zinc causes an excess of copper to accumulate. Supplementing your diet with zinc can help rebalance the situation, but care must be taken to avoid taking too much zinc, which will cause a copper deficiency! It is best to take professional advice before taking large doses of zinc, but a 15mg daily dose is considered quite safe for general use. Zinc has been studied in great detail and a team at the University of Michigan has shown a significant relationship between high academic grades and high zinc levels. Zinc deficiency is prevalent in our society, mainly because of poor soil quality, food processing and bad cooking techniques.

Just like a fire, an epileptic fit starts with a single spark, but the spark in this case is an abnormal brain impulse. The neurotransmitter known as gamma-aminobutyrate acid (GABA) plays a key role in controlling brain impulses. GABA is the most prevalent transmitter in the brain and has many functions, the most important of which is a calming effect on the nervous system. The brains of epileptics, hyperactive children, insomniacs, cerebral palsy sufferers, those suffering from hypertension or anxiety, and those with learning problems, anti-social behaviour and mental retardation, all benefit from elevating GABA levels. GABA has no serious side effects, even in doses of up to 40 grams (the normal dose ranges from 250mcg–1,000mcg daily).

It is interesting to note that zinc again makes an appearance in the natural treatment of epilepsy. Zinc is needed for the production of GABA, along with another amino acid, glutamic acid. Numerous experiments have shown that a zinc-deficient diet aggravates epilepsy and causes more frequent fits and seizures. So far, it can be seen that we need adequate zinc, glutamic acid and vitamin C for the correctly balanced production of neurotransmitters, but the list does not stop there. Vitamin B6 acts as a special co-factor and helps convert the glutamic acid into GABA. If this vitamin is low in the diet, despite adequate amounts of zinc, vitamin C and glutamic acid, the reactions will not occur and GABA levels will fall.

The major structural fats found in the brain are called phospholipids. One particular phospholipid known as phosphatidylserine appears to be important in the control of mood and mood-related problems. Normally this substance is produced naturally in the brain, but in individuals who have deficiencies of vitamin B12, folic acid and other essential fatty acids, the production of phosphatidylserine is dramatically reduced. Low levels are often found in the brains of elderly subjects, but its concentration in younger people may be directly related to depressive mood states.

The primary use of phosphatidylserine in nutritional medicine is in the treatment of depression and impaired mental function in the elderly. Very good results have been obtained in a number of studies (double blind studies). Supplementing the diet with phosphatidylserine appears to improve neurotransmitter release (especially acetylcholine), memory and age-related changes. How phosphatidylserine helps the treatment of depression is unknown. It does not affect serotonin levels like classic antidepressants, nor does it interfere with other neurotransmitters. Phosphatidylserine does, however, improve the quality of brain cell membranes and helps control the levels of cortisol, a hormone released from the adrenal glands that has been found to be elevated in depressed subjects.

All in all, there is much evidence to suggest that the brain needs specific nutrients, and it responds very well to corrective supplements. Feeding your brain well will ensure that it functions optimally and guarantees that long-term deficiency symptoms do not occur. Such symptoms are so slow in developing that they are often written off as being age-related changes for which nothing can be done. This is just not satisfactory, when prevention is so easily achieved by a knowledge of what to feed your brain.

SIX

To Push or Not to Push the Child?

As I have already expressed in this book, I feel increasingly guilty when I think of how bad a father I was at looking after my children. I certainly cared for them in every way possible and I valued the times that I shared with them; cycling, going on day trips and teaching them road safety, but it hurt when one of my daughters once said to me, 'I treasure this park because you took the time to come out with us and have a picnic here.' That actually did not happen often enough. I pushed my children in their education and worked very hard so that I could give them a good future, but sometimes I pushed them too far. One has to be careful to use what my mother used to call 'the golden midway' with children, and look carefully at how much we push them and where we push them. Sometimes we have to leave it to nature. I often see mothers in tears, saying to me, 'I wish my child would work a bit harder' or 'I wish they could concentrate a bit better', because sometimes it is difficult for children to keep up with the pace of life. Other children who take part in adult conversation and television programmes are so wise, and mature so quickly, that they are often shoved in a direction which doesn't benefit them once they go to school.

As I have said, my own brother, Nicolas, was a very good father. He had one handicap. He was slightly dyslexic and my grandmother often said that it was due to her sister (who was a teacher) pushing Nicolas when he was young, because he had a slight stutter. She forced him (as in the old days teachers often did) to overcome this stutter by giving him reading lessons. This is where the mistake was made. She used what we called in Holland the 'reading-board', where you had to put wooden letters in the right place; in those days the key words were '*aap*' (monkey), '*noot*' (nut), '*Mies*' (a name), '*zus*' (sister) and '*Jet*' (another name). My grandmother often said that her sister tried to push and push him to learn to read, and the end result was that she made Nicolas dyslexic, which was, in later life, a big handicap.

It takes a lot of wisdom as the child grows up to know what to do and what not to do. It also sometimes requires a little bit of help. I often watch the three sons of my daughter Maria and son-in-law Marcus, who get very good guidance from their parents, and notice how much the one is influenced by the other. The younger ones will always want to do what the older ones do, but it is all without force. The boys deal with this in a natural way, and I can see how much they learn from interacting and playing with each other.

Then there are children who are very slow, but who have very active parents. The slowness of these children sometimes irritates their parents because they want to push them, which is very often wrong, as this can cause children to become nervous and upset. Sometimes remedies might be of help. I find that if a child's concentration is not too good Concentration Essence, a natural flower essence, might be of benefit. A child's mind can very often wander. Concentration Essence helps with that as its ingredients work mainly on improving the concentration of the mind. As the child grows up, if he or she has difficulties with learning, *Ginkgo biloba* may often be of great help. *Ginkgo biloba* (also known as 'the memory tree') will help activate the brain and will also help the child to memorise things more quickly where extra help is needed.

I also believe, as I mentioned earlier in this book, that cranial osteopathy can often be of some help to children. Cranial osteopathy is a therapy that can help the body to correct or heal itself by a specific technique directed to the bones of the head (the cranium). There are a lot of cranial problems that could influence the magnetism which involves all the bones in the head and spine. To keep a child's back gently working, these movements, which are involuntary, cyclic and essential to the body's line, can be done in every conceivable way.

With a little bit of patience, pushing is not necessary. It is often about sharing the parents' skills with the child, who is possibly more clever than one thinks, and who is often eager to learn, but can sometimes be held back by nerves and anxiety because he or she feels pushed.

It is the same when a child cannot sleep. Why are they crying? Babies always have a reason for crying: they need company, they are hungry, uncomfortable or in pain, or they are bored. A baby who is crying always needs something. It is therefore not a good idea to force the child to sleep. It is better to find out why the child cannot sleep, or why the child does not want to go to bed. Often the child wants to show that it needs some help to sleep, and it can do no harm to give it 15 drops of *Valerian hops*, a gentle herbal remedy which will cause no harm to the child and will help it to sleep. Be careful that you do not over-stimulate the child before bedtime, or stress him or her in any way at all. Try and get the child into bed before he or she gets too tired to sleep, and try to get into a routine that the child likes. Also, listen to any fears that the child might have, as this might be the reason he or she is crying.

It often takes time to discover what your child's needs are, and when you have to let go and when you should give extra encouragement. Children certainly need protection, yet an over-protected child will always lack self-confidence. They will feel threatened when they have to handle challenges on their own. It is the same with obedience. It is absolutely wonderful to teach children to be obedient but, again, children should understand why they should be obedient, and when they need help to do so, you should give children the answers they so badly need to know.

I had a dear friend in the United States who had quite a number of health food shops – big stores of about 25,000 square feet. She had a great love and understanding of children and took a lot of time not only for her own children, but also for others, and she shared a lot of her gifts with children. She used to organise little 'journeys' through her stores for children from a very young age to teenagers, and taught them not only about what to eat and what not to eat, but also about the values of life.

I very often look at her wonderful book, which she personally gave me, entitled *If You Love Me, Don't Feed Me Junk*. She often says that when a child is slow, you should learn the basics of six principles for yourself: Acceptance, Responsibility, Freedom, Honesty, Affirmation and Fun; in order to teach them to a child. She always said you must understand a child before pushing him or her

I like what I once read on the subject of reflective listening, when children are encouraged to be aware, to trust their own feelings and to express their feelings constructively, using reflective listening. Like a mirror, this is meant to reflect the feelings your child is trying to express. Reflecting his or her feelings first of all helps a child to be understood, and it also helps the child to learn the language of feelings. Reflective listening builds the skills needed to understand. Advice was given in the book to establish eye contact, to state the feeling and then define it, and also to slowly help young children with the words when their vocabulary is developing.

I often feel for people when they get frustrated with their children. I tell them to try and keep calm, give it time, and learn to understand the child. A desperate father and mother came to see me last week, both in the teaching profession, who had a child who was growing very slowly. The child was slow both physically and mentally, yet when I performed an iridology and looked deeply into the child's eyes, I knew that there was nothing to worry about. I told the parents to be very careful not to show their child that they were worried about him, as everything would be all right.

There are, however, some good homoeopathic remedies that are very helpful for children who respond slowly. One I have prescribed thousands of times in the 45 years I have been in practice is called *Cerebrum*, because it is often of help if the child needs a little help. If your child is a bit slow to learn, it may also be good to use some reflexology. A reflexologist can easily help with this problem, and in my book *Body Energy* I have outlined various methods to improve, for instance the sucking reflexes of a newborn child (stroking the baby on the cheek makes the baby turn in that direction ready to suck); the grasping reflex (the early grip, which is very strong); the swallowing reflex (practising swallowing fluid in the womb) and the walking reflex, which is lost quickly after birth. There are other reflex therapies that might also be helpful to a child.

This brings me to the different therapies that are good for a pregnant mother when childbirth is imminent, in preparation for labour. Some breathing techniques are very helpful, as are yoga, Alexander technique or pilates. Treating the reflexes is of very great importance and sometimes reflexology can be helpful when the baby is slow in coming. In my book, *Pregnancy and Childbirth*, I have given some advice on this matter.

On diet, we have to realise that in the last 20 years, experts have begun to concede that there might be a number of exceptions to the belief that there is no real malnutrition in Britain. There are the so-called risk groups for whom an otherwise splendid diet might not be enough, and pushing certain foods at children is no good. However, balancing nutrition is the first step – and the most important one – to ensure a sound, structural development when the child grows up. It is very sad that in Britain we still have one of the highest rates of infant deaths and some of the lowest birth weights. Spina bifida, in particular, has a particularly tragic record. Britain has 7,000 cases a year, which is almost the highest in Europe, and in Northern Ireland the rate of 3.4 spina bifida cases per 1,000 is literally the highest for any nation in the world. It is therefore incorrect to say that there is no malnutrition in Britain. There are several books that give information on this subject, as it is important to know what the child needs if he or she is slightly underdeveloped and needs a little encouragement.

Always be receptive, which means listening and being aware when working with children, and also be sensitive to the questions and comments that the child has. Be alert to what is happening around you in nature at the present moment, and focus the child's attention on it without delay. This is most important. I have often said that the first thing that a child sees is a tree. Teach children to become close to nature. In nature everything is in harmony, and children will be very receptive to what is happening around them and will want to get close to nature when they discover flowers and trees.

Children will automatically set out to prove themselves. When they grow up, they will want to run up mountains, to climb and to overcome obstacles. It is therefore important for the child to learn the sounds of nature, and see the colours and the light. A child should learn about the natural world of animals. It is important that when children grow up, we see these things through their eyes as they develop.

As for all the parents I have seen in the past who were so worried that their child wasn't growing quickly enough, I cannot stress enough how important it is that the child learns to eat the right foods and be surrounded by nature as much as possible. It is also important that as children grow up they eat the right grains. It might be a good idea to invest in organic grains. The chromosomes in organically grown grains are very much lower than they are in grains that are developed in artificial manure and treated with insecticides, pesticides and fertilisers. Food is extremely important for the child's growth, especially when parents want to push their child into a faster growing pattern. Some very good research work has been done into children's nutrition and the benefits of grains. Breakfast is terribly important. I still remember a time when Dr Vogel and I sent 40 children into the mountains for a 15-mile walk up a hill and a 15-mile walk back down, on a plate of muesli mixed with the juice of an orange, a grated apple and some banana. They came back hungry, but not exceptionally hungry, because that breakfast had provided them with good nutrition for the day.

Supporting the UK's leading nutrition experts in the WGFH campaign, celebrity Gloria Hunniford said: 'Like most of us, I lead a really busy life, juggling career and family and, as I get older, I concentrate more and more on eating a balanced diet with lots of unrefined foods to help me keep healthy and full of vitality. This new information on whole grain shows that simple changes, such as adding wholegrain cereal or bread to our daily diet, can have a significant health benefit. I am certainly going to go with the grain and encourage my friends and family to enjoy these great benefits too.'

Whole grain means that all parts of the grain are used: the fibre-rich bran (outer layer), the endosperm (middle layer) and the nutrient-packed germ (inner layer). Previously, it was thought that whole grain reduced the risk of disease because it is a good source of fibre, but recent research confirms that the 'wholegrain package' (including its other components: antioxidants, vitamins, minerals, complex carbohydrates and phytochemicals) protects the body against many diseases. However, the WGFH survey findings revealed that a staggering 93 per cent of respondents thought that only the fibre content of whole grain was responsible for its health benefits.

'The evidence is compelling that a diet rich in wholegrain foods has a protective effect against several forms of cancer and heart disease,' says Dr Susan Jebb, Head of Nutrition and Health Research at the Medical Research Council's Human Nutrition Unit. 'This disease-preventing capability is not solely due to the dietary fibre found in whole grain. The whole grain delivers abundant amounts of antioxidant vitamins and phytochemicals that appear to act together to provide protective effects.'

Wholegrain foods are classified as foods that contain 51 per cent or more wholegrain ingredients, such as wholegrain wheat or oats, so whole grain will always be the first ingredient listed on the packet. Breakfast cereals (such as porridge oats) and wholemeal breads (such as Hovis Wholemeal) provide the bulk of whole grain in the UK, as well as wholegrain rice and pasta products. In the nationwide WGFH survey, 72 per cent of Brits say that they now want more wholegrain foods in their diet, but 77 per cent do not currently check whether the food they purchase contains whole grain, and up to 80 per cent admit they are confused about which foods are actually made with whole grain.

'Sometimes people think they're eating a wholegrain food, but often they are not. Just because a bread looks dark doesn't necessarily mean it is made with whole grain,' explains Maryon Stewart, Founder and Director of the Women's Nutritional Advisory Service. 'It is important to check the ingredient list – the first ingredient should always be a whole grain or wholemeal, such as "wholegrain oats", "wholemeal flour", "wholegrain wheat" or "whole wheat".'

In addition to protecting against heart disease, research has shown that eating wholegrain foods is associated with a reduced risk of the following cancers: colonic, rectum, gastric, endometrial, oral, pharyngeal, tongue and oesophageal. 'With approximately 200,000 new cancer cases emerging each year and the highest incidence in Europe, it is vital that we do all we can to reduce these numbers. There is now a clear scientific consensus that cancers are largely preventable, with dietary changes, such as including whole grain, playing an important role,' explained a source from the Cancer Research/Support Organisation.

University of Minnesota epidemiologist Dr David R. Jacobs, who has published numerous studies on the health benefits of whole grain, has even more extensive data. 'Our research shows that those who habitually ate wholegrain products each day had about a 15 to 25 per cent reduction in death from all causes, including heart disease and cancer.' In his research, Dr Jacobs speculates that if people ate at least one serving of whole grain each day, deaths from heart disease and cancer in the overall population could be cut by 8 per cent. Just under 300,000 Brits currently die from heart disease and cancer every year. An 8 per cent decrease in deaths from these diseases would translate to approximately 24,000 lives saved each year.

The Food and Drugs Administration (FDA) last year authorised a new health claim to promote the heart disease-fighting and cancer-fighting health benefits of wholegrain foods. 'Diets rich in wholegrain foods and other plant foods and low in total fat, saturated fat and cholesterol, may reduce the risk of heart disease and some cancers.' American dietary guidelines recently published by four national health organisations, including the American Heart Association and American Cancer Society, recommended the consumption of at least three wholegrain servings per day. The WGFH survey shows that only 15 per cent of the British population currently eat three servings per day of wholegrain cereals or bread.

This report is interesting, as I personally feel that children have a much better chance when they have eaten the right kind of food, which provides the nutrition they need to push them in the right direction and prepare them for life.

SEVEN

To Work or Not to Work?

Women today are fortunate to be able to choose to work. Even 50 years ago, this was often simply not an option. Women's lives were mapped out for them; it was expected that they would get married, have children and look after the home. Not to have achieved this was often seen as a failure.

Times have changed. A historical, long and hard campaign earned the right for women to follow other options, with many women choosing to have a career before settling down to family life. It is then that hard decisions have to be made – to work or not to work? Or is there a happy medium? Modern equipment removes the need to have each day mapped out with specific chores. The washing and ironing can be pushed to the end of the day, leaving the rest of the day for other, higher priorities. Is this time going to be spent with the children and looking after the home, or is part of it or the majority of it going to be spent working?

Women have a few months during the end of their pregnancy and the first few months of their babies' lives to make the huge decision whether or not they are going to return to work. The options are certainly there, but which is the best? The answer to this is that there is no best option, simply what suits the situation at the time. Mothers have to question both what they want and what they need from work and home life. Do they need to work to pay for the basic bills or for the little extras, for their personal self-fulfilment, or simply because their careers form a high priority? The next consideration is how it will affect the family unit, as well as the mother's own health and energy.

Most women would agree that there is an element of guilt involved with combining work and family. If the reasons why you work are clear, then there is little point in feeling guilty. If you can't change the situation, this negative emotion will clearly affect the children. They will quickly pick up on your emotions, even subconsciously, and behave in ways that will make you feel even guiltier. You then run the risk of spoiling the children to compensate for the guilt. There are other factors which can increase this feeling. If you are merely working to meet the general materialistic pressures of modern life, then the sense of inadequacy this reveals needs to be addressed. In this case you are sure to feel guilty for working (subconsciously you know that these extras are unnecessary and that your child would rather have your love and company than another new toy), but worse than that is the fact that this bowing down to peer pressure is sure to leave you dissatisfied with your lot in life. How many people do you know who, once they have purchased the car of their dreams, are already looking for a 'better' one or, having bought a house, are counting the years until they buy a bigger one? Most of us have this feeling of wanting to reach a particular goal – it's natural and is called achieving. But is it really necessary to have these things for personal fulfilment, or would you lead a happier life without the pressure of work – a little poorer perhaps, but able to give the rare commodity of time to your family?

The full-time homemaker is becoming rare, with many women choosing to work full- or, more commonly, part-time. Sadly, it's a known fact that the majority of housewives simply do not feel their own self-worth. We have noted in the clinics that when the receptionist questions the occupation when filling out the initial details on the client's case history form, the reply of 'I'm *just* a housewife' is frequent. To see this illustrated, you need look no further than 'picking up' time from school at the end of the day. There is a definite distinction between the working mums and the homemakers, each denouncing the other. Why do so many women feel that they have to justify what they do, and why do the homemakers, who choose to do a worthwhile and important job, feel this way? If they have answered the question as to why they have chosen their lifestyle, there should be no need for justification or guilt. They are doing what is needed and is best for, firstly, their family and, secondly, to meet the basic need of survival.

The majority of women return to work at some point after having children and half do so before their children start school. So what are the options for a working mum, and who looks after the children in her absence?

Whether you choose a part-time or full-time situation, it is clear that a strong support network is essential. For the high-flyer, one of the most successful methods is to swap roles. Many years ago it would have been virtually unheard of for fathers to look after the children and home. In this century we shall see many more fathers adopting this role. Mostly this occurs by change of circumstance and not by planning. Perhaps the father has been made redundant, or his wife has better job prospects. With so many successful career women and with equal rights (more or less) in the workplace, dads at home is certainly an option, and they often find it more fulfilling than women whose careers may have come to an abrupt halt. Again, it boils down to what you want from life.

The next option most people consider is family to help care for their children, and usually this responsibility is put to grandmothers, who tend to fall into two definite categories – those who want to be involved and those who don't. There are two drawbacks to family as child-carers. One is that the mother has to accept advice (often unwanted) from a relative. The other is the reliability factor. Family members have their own lives and although the idea of looking after a little tot may be appealing initially, this option will simply not work if the novelty wears off after a few months; it may be carers find that the children encroach too much into their social situations. From the outset, there has to be a clear understanding by both parties of what is expected from each other, both must sympathise with each other's needs and the mother must never take the carer for granted. This may mean, for instance, forgoing the social aspect of work (the after-work drinks and functions).

Working from home seems a great ideal if possible. But again there are drawbacks. Depending on what you do, there may be work demands that simply do not fit in with those of your child. There will come a time when the baby's morning and afternoon naps become less frequent, teething will upset him or her, or boredom may simply set in and your attention will be required. Will it be possible to cope with telephone calls and deadlines when you are torn between two priorities?

The other option involves help from an outside source. A childminder is the most affordable option, where you drop your child off at the minder's house and pick them up after work. Day-care nurseries are becoming a common option, where you drop off your child and pick him or her up at a designated time. Some workplaces even provide their own day-care nurseries for their workers' children. Probably the most expensive, but most flexible option, is a nanny who comes to your home. Over the years, nannies have received much bad press, but it is worth bearing in mind that often these nightmare stories are based on an initial bad choice. Everyone has their own individual views on the best way to bring up children and, from the outset, it is the parents' duty to find a nanny who reflects their own ideas to avoid conflict. There also has to be mutual respect. After all, they are responsible for your nearest and dearest in your absence.

Successful communication of what you expect from the start will benefit everyone, especially the child. Each of the above options for childcare has its benefits and drawbacks. There are many stories of the successes and failures of each method. It is up to the parents to weigh up the pros and cons and even go by their instinct as to what would suit their own unique situation. To feel comfortable with your choice is paramount. There is little point in returning to work if you spend most of your time checking up and hanging on the phone to see what is going on with the child.

Few people will argue that children make demands on your energy. The amount of planning and organisation increases as children's needs are taken into consideration. There is no doubt that life does become more complicated and, with the extra worries that children bring, parents' own health becomes of prime importance. You have to be strong and healthy in order to look after the children and home effectively. Sleep is one of the most important commodities. When children arrive on the scene, it is best to forget the late evenings and 'burning the candle at both ends'. Bed and sleep become precious, leaving the majority of parents adopting an 'early to bed' attitude for themselves. Some time alone is essential, especially if you work. You need to set a little time aside for something you enjoy. Whether this is a game of tennis or a relaxing bath, it is important to try and arrange childcare, even for a short time, to allow yourself a break, if not each day, certainly every week. Children do not cope well with frazzled, anxious parents.

Taking to bed with a cold or flu is simply not an option for most mothers. They tend to barge on regardless, leaving their own immune system depleted. As a preventative, a good diet, with regular meals (which includes at least five portions of fruit and vegetables daily) is beneficial. If you feel you are a little low, take an additional immune booster, such as *Echinacea* or *Beta glucan*, along with a multivitamin which includes vitamin C and the B vitamins. If you do fall ill or feel under the weather and there is no one to take over the childcare responsibilities, prioritise. Leave the pile of ironing for another day; instead of doing rigorous activities with your child, choose calmer ones such as reading or drawing. When your children rest or sleep, you should also use this time to lie down and take a nap.

Regardless of whether you choose to work or not, there is no doubt that children are hard work and require an infinite amount of attention. There is no easy option, but when the going gets tough, keep the basic principles in mind. Your children are the priority, and the reason you chose your lifestyle probably revolved around their needs. So when you feel stressed, whether it has been a hard day at work, the children themselves have been difficult or you have other worries, remember that it is not your child's fault. If there are problems surrounding the child, come to terms with them and do what you can to sort the difficulties out and, above all, always keep the child's needs at heart, even if this requires more effort on your behalf.

Balance is the key. Sometimes the decisions you will need to make may be tough on the children and, when this occurs, you can support them and be there, always listening to their needs. But remember, there are times when you cannot give your child everything that he or she wants, and although this may be hard for everyone, it can be beneficial to them. Children need to know about boundaries, and they need to understand why you work. By giving them this understanding, you will not have to compensate for your lack of time with gifts – they will know that you are doing it for them. Above all, you will be setting an example for their future. As the years go by, life for growing children becomes harder. The pressure starts for them from the moment they start school, and it continues from there, with a lot of competition in the job market. Few children have the luxury of having life given to them on a plate. People have to work hard at who they are and children need to be encouraged at a young age to develop the skills of promoting their personalities, building on their good points and keeping their negative points in check.

Supportive parenting is the key, and if you make enough time for your child (remember quality time is better than quantity time) his or her future should not be affected, whether you work or not.

EIGHT

Hyperactivity and Allergies

The other day, during a busy practice at my clinic, a mother came in with her child who, in no time, had wrecked both the waiting-room and the hall. Everyone was in fear and trembling as the child ran loose like a wild animal. The child was bashing the furniture, took a stick and knocked on the big, old standing clock, threw itself on the floor and screamed. I decided to take the mother and the child quickly into a consulting room. It wasn't long before I saw that the poor child was in torment because of hyperactivity.

There are lots of books written on hyperactive children, with much advice being given but, again, it needed a lot of understanding to find out why this poor child became hyperactive. Very often, hyperactive children are allergic to sugar, additives or colouring and when these are cut out of the diet, life can become easier. This particular child was swearing at the mother, uttering appalling language. I felt very, very sorry for the poor child. On another occasion, the same mother had been found crying because her child was swearing at her. I told the mother that the lollipop the child was waving around wouldn't do it a lot of good and I researched the child's daily diet. I then simply asked her if she wanted the child to be treated my way, and if she would cooperate. That child is now a delightful creature who has changed totally within two months. Thankfully, this child is now loving and most appreciative to have finally been freed from this horrendous torment. This child didn't want to behave in this way, but simply couldn't help it. Nutrition has so much to do with mind and behaviour, and one of my books, *Nutrition and Mental Behaviour*, explains this.

It is very often the case that if the hyperactive child is not treated properly and has an unhealthy diet, then that child can grow up to be an uncontrollable youngster. I once interviewed the mother of one of my life-sentence prisoners (I go to prisons to study the mental behaviour, hyperactivity and allergies of prisoners and what their childhood was like). His mother was wonderful and loving, but I asked her what she gave her little son to keep him quiet when he was uncontrollable. The answer was chocolate, sweeties – the lot. That was the only thing that would make her son behave. In all her loving kindness, she didn't know that she was bringing up a boy who would become a criminal and a murderer. That same man who, in his youth, didn't get the treatment he should have, became a different character when his diet was looked at properly. Nowadays in our clinics, we have machines where we can test for food allergies and this fellow, when I tested him, had five different allergies – wheat, milk, sugar, coffee and bread – all the things he was eating when he committed murder. I cannot stress enough in this book how important it is that parents investigate their children's allergies when they become hyperactive and see that they receive treatment.

In February 1993, a two-year-old child, Jamie Bulger, was abducted from a shopping centre in the north of England and brutally abused and murdered. The most shocking aspect of the tragedy was that the killers were two ten-year-old boys and the whole nation was horrified as more details unfolded. There was a great public debate about the case and the boys were punished by the justice system. In the media there was much discussion about violence and abuse, the breakdown of families and poverty in Britain. All this caused a great deal of food for thought. Why did the two boys murder this two-year-old child? There were a lot of theories put forward as to why this particular incident happened, but often it is children who are brought up on the wrong kind of foods, becoming addicted to lemonade and sweets at a very young age, who cause trouble. When visiting prisons where I have interviewed men and women on this subject, I have often asked myself the question, 'Where has society failed?' Slowly, we have become a selfish society where there is a tendency to think 'As long as I'm all right, Jack, the rest can do what they like.'

I saw in the paper a very cruel murder that took place in a

tenement in Glasgow. Several people passed by and didn't do a single thing to help the little old lady who was monstrously murdered. Where is the care that we should have for others? Where is the care that we should have for children? Where is the love that we should have for life? It all comes back to a question asked in the Bible. Cain murdered his brother Abel. When God enquired about this, Cain answered, 'Am I my brother's keeper?' It is very sad that our society has become so selfish that we don't care for each other any more. There is a great injustice if we do not learn to share our life with others, and certainly if we don't give it to our children.

Hyperactivity in children is a very big problem today and can often be cured. My uncle, who was the head of a psychiatric hospital in Holland with 2,500 mentally handicapped patients, often asked me when I was studying to help out with organising festivities in the hospital. It always amazed me how many of these people tucked into chocolates, biscuits and other sugary products. Sugar is one of the biggest addictions that one can have. My ex-criminal friend, who carried out many murders, is now a happy man and has great respect for the foods he is allergic to. A lot could therefore be done with dietary management. Foods which affect one's mental state so much can be greatly reduced so that they will not affect one's mind. I often speak in my books of a 'low stress diet', or a diet that has a good balance of protein and carbohydrate. This balance is necessary in order to keep one's mind fresh and more adjusted to dealing with daily living.

The child who becomes hyperactive and breaks things to pieces certainly needs help. A lot of problems with hyperactivity have emerged since our diets have changed in modern times and much can be done to help parents understand the hyperactivity problem, which can be helped so much with good food management. As children get older they have 'growth spurts', when they have tremendous nutritional demand. They need more vitamins and, although they will have their own favourite foods, it is important that their staple diet at home stresses the importance of adequate vitamins and minerals. It is very sad to see what can happen to their health and mental well-being if they do not get these vitamins and minerals. There is more information on this subject in Chapter Twelve.

I feel so sorry for the younger generation when I see addiction to alcohol and drugs growing steadily and, as a father and grandfather, I held my heart the other day when I came out of the railway station and saw three teenage girls, between the ages of 15 and 17, lying in the street, totally drunk. They were completely unable even to cross the road in the state they were in. One could see in their faces how deficient they were and the foods they needed. I asked myself the question, 'Is this the future?' Don't we have a duty to try harder to meet the needs of these children, and give them better support in order to protect not only their physical health, but also their minds? The mind is stronger than the body, and they all need a strong mental and physical immunity to help them with today's threats to their health. I personally feel that I have to do a lot more to help those youngsters when they grow up, to try and show them that there is a healthier way of living and that one can get a lot more out of life in doing so.

There are all kinds of allergies. When I graduated in 1968, there was only a small selection of books on allergies. There are now so many books on allergies that they would fill a whole church, and yet no one really understands the allergy problem properly. It is possible to cut out wheat, milk, sugar and alcohol, and yet still be allergic. It depends a lot on the immune system, and the strength of the immune system will often determine how bad an allergy is. Often colleagues have come into my treatment rooms and asked me how I treat allergies. I tell them I treat the immune system. Once the immune system is treated, I look at the remaining allergies, and then I treat that problem. It is very important that we look first at how the immune system copes with the allergic reactions.

After the immune system has been treated, there are wonderful remedies which can be used to desensitise the body to the allergy, such as *Harpagophytum* (devil's claw), and a powerful remedy from the States called 'ALR', produced by a company called Michaels, which desensitises certain allergies.

I once asked one of my best friends, a great immunologist, if he understood the problem of allergies, and he said, 'Do you understand it?' We both agreed how difficult it was to understand allergies, as we basically don't know exactly how the immune system works. He is an expert on the subject, has written many books about it and can tell us about the A-lymphocytes, the B-lymphocytes and the T-lymphocytes with very sophisticated evidence, and yet he too is often surprised when he sees how the immune system works, and how allergies very often rotate when the immune system is low and needs building up.

With hyperactive children, I often get good results from asking them to cut out sugar, coloured lemonades and additives, and add some flower essences, like Child Essence (a wonderful flower essence to help the hyperactive child) or even *Avena sativa* (the extract of fresh oats). This treatment can calm the child beautifully.

In general, allergies can be treated if we are willing to go on a diet to try and find out what leads to allergic reactions. I once saw a very hyperactive child who was scratching to ease what a doctor had said was an unidentified skin disease. The child was frantic and couldn't cope. She nearly scratched her head off with the terrible itching. The child was certainly addicted to a few foods. The foods she was eating that had a bad effect on her were the ones she was most fond of, as is often the case. Yet when I started to cut these foods out of her diet, she got better and better, and was soon almost a new character. It is often a question of finding out exactly what is happening.

How do we understand allergies? As my friend the immunologist said, 'It is a question of research and continuing to look for the answer as to where an allergy might have occurred or has developed because of certain circumstances.' In my book *Viruses, Allergies and the Immune System*, I have given much evidence of allergic reactions that one can develop due to things one comes into contact with, and one has to be very careful. If foods cause an allergic reaction, cut these foods out – even temporarily – so that one can find out where the allergies come from.

Why does someone suddenly develop a milk or dairy food allergy? I am often asked that question. Is milk or cheese so bad? Cows' milk can form mucus and if a person is allergic to it, then goats' milk is a good alternative. I do find that if a child is sensitive to cows' milk, goats' milk is usually safe. It has a different effect on the body. The level of protein in goats' milk is around 2.9 per cent (compared with cows' milk at 3.3 per cent). While this substantial protein content is needed by the rapidly growing calf, it is excessive for human children and the extra protein can stress the infant's liver and kidneys. The protein level in this formula is reduced to 1.4 per cent, a value in keeping with the infant's needs.

Also very important is the fact that the casein in goats' milk is quite different: where both cows' and goats' milk contain alpha casein, beta casein and kappa casein, goats' milk contains no gamma casein, which is so prominent in cows' milk. There is no major cross-reactivity between the caseins of the two species. The alpha casein in cows' milk is alpha-1s, whereas in goats' milk it is alpha-2s. The difference between the casein is emphasised by goats' milk casein only having half the potency of cows' milk. Therefore, goats' milk protein compares well with human milk protein in the amino acid composition. The fat content of goats' milk is also different to that of cows' milk. Therefore, when there are certain allergies, the food that can be used instead often has a better action and the allergy should be well understood and possibly, with a little bit of guidance, lead to better food management. Allergies can lead to a lot of problems with infections and therefore both hyperactivity and allergies should be treated and not neglected.

Infections were formerly the most frequent causes of disease. In our time, allergies (mainly from food) are increasing uncontrollably. Over 70 per cent of the population of the industrial countries have an allergic disposition. Allergies are 'new' diseases which in the past were hardly known. All the illnesses I call 'civilisation diseases' are caused principally by our modern Western lifestyle and nutritional habits, as well as by the pollution of our environment.

When speaking of an allergy, we mean a *changed or unusual defensive reaction against specific well-known or unknown substances*. An allergic disposition can be hereditary or acquired. An allergic reaction to a substance or to food can happen within seconds or over a period of up to 72 hours. Innumerable health problems or even serious illness can be caused by allergens. Most affected are the skin and the mucous membranes. There is no need to describe here the very complicated process that can trigger off an allergic reaction. What we want to know is *why* we actually become allergic.

Until about 100 years ago, an allergy was something out of the ordinary. Now it is officially accepted that the contamination of our modern environment has created a climate propitious for the development of such illnesses. We can get an allergy at any time in life, even as early as a bottle-fed baby. The organism of the baby has been intended for the digestion of mothers' milk, which has a completely different quality and composition from cows' milk. As I have explained, a baby cannot completely assimilate and digest cows' milk or any milk other than mothers' milk, even if this has been altered in order to resemble human milk. In such 'alien' milk, there are always foreign substances that cannot be digested or eliminated, and the organism of the baby must somehow get rid of these, as they interfere with many internal procedures.

The easiest way for the organism to excrete these substances is through the skin and, in this case, the baby will suffer from all kinds of skin problems, such as the so-called 'milk crust'. If these skin problems are not treated correctly or if the symptoms are suppressed by medication, very often more serious diseases may develop and the baby retains an allergic disposition throughout its entire life. It will be extremely sensitive to all kinds of allergens, not only to those from milk and milk products.

At the beginning of the 20th century, there were only a few food additives on the market; nowadays there are thousands of them, as well as innumerable foreign substances in the environment. It is logical that the human organism tries to defend itself against all these toxins. Even when a certain substance is harmless in itself, it is possible that through its combination with other additives, new and often very toxic substances can come into being. In medicine these dangers are known, and many books have been written on this subject, but the threat is completely ignored by the food industry.

Not only industrial products, but also natural products can contain allergens from agriculture or cattle breeding. One can have an allergic reaction to almost anything, and such a reaction can take place in any form, in any part of the body. An allergic disposition can be dormant for many years and break out only after the person in question comes into contact with certain allergens while his defensive forces are under par. The first signs of an allergy may be headaches, dizziness or migraine headaches that occur more or less regularly. People suffering from bronchitis, sinusitis or asthma often owe their disease to an allergic disposition. The same applies in the case of tachycardia (rapid heartbeat), shortage of breath and similar problems. Mothers, especially during pregnancy, should seek medical guidance if they are having any of these allergic reactions. After being breast-fed and going over to cows' milk, babies often suffer from eczema. If this is the case, they should be given goats' milk or soya milk instead.

If the cause of the allergy can be discovered and removed, it is often surprising how quickly many health problems disappear. But most of the time it is very difficult to find these so-called 'allergens' (substances which trigger off allergic reactions in the body). An allergic reaction can be caused by an addiction to certain kinds of food. If, for example, a person loves chocolate and eats it every day, or almost every day, certain defensive reactions against the very concentrated contents such as refined sugar, industrial cocoa, saturated fats etc. in these products become overstrained and it becomes impossible for the organism to replace the specific defensive cells needed quickly enough. In this case the body has to take other measures, and any part of the body will cooperate in order to defend itself against these allergens.

This situation can be compared with an army. When a particular unit is unable to continue to fight, other units have to take over. The next battle might then be fought somewhere else, with different weapons. The same thing happens in the human body, and far more diseases than we presently realise are caused by allergens; that is by certain substances with which the body can no longer cope.

Unfortunately, most doctors do not understand this and they treat, for example, an asthmatic reaction or bronchitis with medication that suppresses the symptoms. That the patient in question could be, for example, allergic to cows' milk, sugar, chocolate or certain chemical substances in food is completely ignored. Because of this, millions of patients have to take suppressive medication throughout their lives. If your child has such chronic health problems, you should try to cut out of his or her diet for one or two weeks any food which he or she eats regularly. It is very possible that health problems will disappear completely when the offensive substance is taken away. Any child who gets allergic reactions after eating his or her favourite food should refrain from having it in the future. If there is a wheat allergy, rye, barley or millet is a good alternative. If your child has a nut allergy, you should be very careful that he or she does not come into contact with any food containing nuts, as it can be very dangerous.

Allergic problems can also be traced by watching a change in behaviour pattern. Often, it is not the food itself but the additives in the food that cause allergies. In that case, it is easy to explain why people are not always allergic to the same food, but to certain brands. If there are no additives in the food, there will be no allergic reactions.

ALLERGIES AND MENTAL DISEASE

Formerly, hardly anybody would have thought that mental diseases, physical problems, or unusual behaviour could have anything to do with food allergies. This changed when some doctors in North America, England, and later in Germany, started to look into these problems. Scientists such as Ted Randolph, Herbert Rinkel, Albert Rowe, George Watson, Professor Comrey, Richard Mackarness, Professor Pfister, Lothar Burgerstein, Anna Calantin, along with many others, achieved outstanding results in this field.

It also became known that Hippocrates (460 BC) and other famous doctors of antiquity treated people who were mentally ill with laxatives, emetics and special diets with much success. They were convinced that mental diseases and abnormal behaviour were often caused by a malfunction of the metabolism and not by a *sick mind* or a *bad or unbalanced personality*. Some American physicians proved, as far back as 50 years ago, that a criminal mind can often be linked to *wrong nutritional habits* and to *some specific foods*. They found out that many criminals lived almost exclusively on so-called junk food or fast food, and ate fried chicken with French fries regularly, often cooked in the same old oil which had been reheated many times.

Old, rancid oil is not only a vitamin and mineral robber, but it can also damage and paralyse brain or nerve cells. Many criminals often react like zombies, as if they are in a kind of trance and do not really know what is going on.

It is quite interesting that some hyperactive children often behave in a similar way. Of course, rancid oil is not the only culprit but, in combination with other refined and unnatural foods, it will be harmful not only for the body, but also for the mind.

FOODS WHICH CAN TRIGGER OFF ALLERGIES

More and more people are allergic to milk and dairy products. Different kinds of cereal (especially wheat), refined carbohydrates, eggs, citrus fruits (mainly when they have been sprayed or waxed), tomatoes, chocolate, sausages, pork, breakfast cereals and tinned food can also cause allergic reactions.

If you suspect that you might be allergic to a food you eat quite often, you should cut it out of your diet for four or five days and then try a little on an empty stomach in the morning. If you get a negative reaction, like a headache or a rapid heartbeat, this is a sign that you should no longer eat this food.

In this way you can test many different kinds of food, and find out which causes an allergic reaction. This method is practised in hospitals and clinics which specialise in treating food allergies; the only difference is that for the first few days the patients are put on a so-called 'water fast'. During this time they are not allowed to eat anything; they must drink only water, so that their digestive tract will become as clean as possible.

PHOSPHATES IN THE FOOD

It is interesting, because of the many additives and artificial colourings used today, how many mothers and children have allergic reactions – the number seems to be increasing all the time. Some of the food additives used most frequently today are phosphates, which are considered harmless by the authorities provided that the daily intake is no more than 750mg.

Phosphates really can do miracles. They can make dull, unattractive, old and wilted food look fresh and appetising, and are used in the cheese and meat industry, in manufacturing cakes, pastries, soups, sauces, chocolate, soft drinks, etc. They have excellent qualities as buffers, emulsifiers, thickening agents, coagulators, water absorbers and for rendering certain substances inactive. Foods which children like best are embellished and improved by phosphates in order to make them more attractive: sausages, hamburgers, soft drinks, ice cream, pastries, sweets, puddings and so on – all of them contain phosphates. Therefore, children often eat more than twice the amount recommended for adults.

Symptoms of an overdose of phosphates are often quite serious; one, for example, is MCD (minimal cerebral dysfunction).

Other symptoms are:

(a) Hyperactivity, hypoactivity and autism. Hyperactive children fidget all the time and never keep quiet. Hypoactive and autistic children, on the other hand, have lost all *joie de vivre* and seem to have no energy at all.

(b) Antisocial behaviour.

(c) Disturbed muscular functions and uncontrolled movements.

(d) Congenital alexia: children with spelling and reading problems.

(e) Lack of concentration, children cannot listen.

(f) Fear of physical contact.

(g) Osteoporosis: disorders of bone healing.

(h) Pylorus cramps: cramps of the stomach muscles.

(i) Pseudo croup: coughing fits because of restricted air passage.

(j) Disorders of the heart muscle.

(k) Allergies: asthma, hay fever, nettle rash, eczema.

(l) Different skin diseases, e.g. neurodermatitis.

(m) Vasomotoric disorders, e.g. migraine. Disorders of stomach and intestinal dysfunctions, stomach ulcers, ulcers of the duodenum.

Herta Hafer, the author of the book *The Secret Drug – Food Phosphate,* presents readers with many sound arguments and proof of this.

There has been much scientific research done on this subject, but for several reasons most of this has not been published or is simply ignored. Certainly, not all of the symptoms mentioned above come only from an overdose of phosphates, and every disease has more than one cause, but it is time to research this situation more thoroughly.

NINE

Autism

About 20 years ago Prof. Roger McDougall and I went to a well-known university. A professor there wanted to ask us our views on gluten. We spoke to this professor and I distinctly remember that Prof. Roger McDougall spoke about schizophrenia and autism. He went so far as to say that autistic children were allergic to gluten and possibly to casein. The professor very kindly nodded his head, but we were quickly removed from the university, as I am sure he thought we were two nutcases. On a later visit to another university we were met with the same attitude, and I can only say that over the years, when Roger spoke on his well-known gluten-free diets, he was met with very little understanding.

How the world has changed. Today, when we read scientific papers from universities all over the world, we now often see autism referred to as an allergy to gluten and to casein. Poor Roger McDougall, who is dead and gone now, never saw the fruits of his labour. He worked so hard to convince the world of his convictions, based on his own situation; he was almost blind and unable to walk, but after he cut out gluten from his diet, he not only got his sight back, but also regained his mobility and could walk even faster than I.

Over the years, I have looked into the gluten debate from several angles. I have seen that with schizophrenia we often have positive results from cutting out gluten, and I have also had great results in helping parents reverse the effects autism has had on their children. Sometimes when I look at these children, some of whom focus, while others don't, I am really very sorry for them, because some of these wonderful, good-looking children have been transported into a world which is not their own. Autism is so very misunderstood.

The British psychiatrist Lorna Wing believes in two types of impairment – underlying and secondary. Although not all authorities agree with her, the distinction is indeed very helpful. Symptoms of autism include language problems, abnormalities, facial expressions, abnormal responses, motor control problems, secondary impairments, aloofness, routine problems, emotional reactions, imagination, immaturity and problems making sense of things. We talk sometimes about classic autism or autistic features and although not all autistic children show these personalities or characteristics, the onset of autism is a very frightening one.

What worries me most is that I see autism growing and there are more cases now than I have ever seen before. I therefore feel that diet has a lot to do with the condition. The general bowel control studies conducted in hospitals and research have really failed to show the abnormality of the child or what the causes could be. It can be a combination of brain damage, slight abnormality or shock. Again, parents are very important in treating the autistic child. The management of the disease, education and future outlook of the children depend a lot on how they develop when they receive treatment.

I often find, when I look at the kind of birth an autistic child has had, that this plays a very big role. Sometimes when the birth has been difficult, and often when forceps have been used, the child might have a little cranial damage and, in some autistic children, carrying out cranial osteopathy to balance the cranium has been beneficial. However, the best results I have had were with a completely gluten-free diet, keeping sugar very low, and with no casein. I also use a few remedies – some vitamins, minerals and trace elements from Michaels and *Cerebrum* in homoeopathy, which I have found to be very effective.

I saw a young boy of five the other day. He was completely uncontrollable and lived totally in his own world. He could not concentrate, but after he had treatment his mother told me that his teacher had said how well he was coming on. This was a most surprising and wonderful result, giving this boy the skills that were necessary for him to cope with life. It is wonderful to see how much can be done for children with autism, although when one witnesses a real autism case, one realises how much one has to do.

According to the National Autistic Society (NAS), all those with autism have impairment in social interaction, social communication and imagination. These traits make autistic children appear aloof and indifferent. They are also unable to interpret facial expressions and tones of voice and have a limited range of play activities, possibly copied and pursued repetitively. Autism is often referred to as 'autistic spectrum disorder'. NAS suggest that there are around 500,000 people with autism spectrum disorders in the UK. It affects over 90 people in every 10,000 of the population and seems to be increasing. Its increase is also apparent in other countries.

There are many suggestions as to why autism is so much on the increase. Personally, I feel that poor nutrition is one of the reasons. Certainly, inoculations might be a cause, but nobody is sure. How far the MMR vaccine can be proven to be linked to autism is still in question. What is interesting is that males with autism outnumber females by four to one.

Children with autism have raised levels of immune system markers – high levels of serotonin (the brain chemical associated with sleep, mood and depression) – and researchers are looking further into nutritional deficiencies. Researchers at the University of Birmingham have found that around 95 per cent of autistic children have low levels of a substance needed to deactivate the key neurotransmitters (the nervous system's chemical messengers) involved in the behaviour of mood, and believe that linoleic acids may have an involvement in this. A complete antioxidant will reduce toxins and waste material within an autistic child's body. With autism, you have to look carefully at the diet (which might need some improvement), carry out a detoxification, and observe the child's behaviour and reactions carefully. Once put on a diet and introduced to remedies such as *Cerebrum*, *Child Essence* and possibly a full spectrum of vitamins, minerals and trace elements, available both for boys and girls from Michaels, help can often be given. Sometimes when the immune system is very low, I advocate *Super Immuno Comp*, an excellent remedy from Enzymatic, which is of great help in the child's immunity.

Autism frequently goes unnoticed at birth, but as the child grows and certain characteristics appear, it is necessary to look at how the five senses work to ensure that they are developing as they should. There might be some problems. As I have often said, when you lose your senses, you lose your sense of living. Always keep an eye on touch, smell, vision, hearing and taste. These will be the first things that will appear to be abnormal in autism and give cause for concern. In my book *The Five Senses*, I have given a lot of examples on how to deal with that. There are some children for whom I had little hope, but when I look at how some of them have developed under the guidance of their parents, I am very happy that the advice that the parents took from me has been so beneficial for their child.

Dead foods (foods which are not natural and fresh) will be of no use to the autistic child. Their immunity and growth process depends a great deal on what kind of food we give them to eat and remedies we help them with. It is good to help concentrate the child's mind, as I saw with one mother who taught her autistic child to blow soap bubbles in the air. She learned to concentrate better and with the help of *Cerebrum* and *Child Essence* – and what I call 'living' foods – the child now leads a normal life.

LIVING AND DEAD FOODS

What is really meant by 'living' foods is very important, as a large part of our modern diet has become, as Prof. Kollath often said, 'dead' food, which has been killed by different manipulations and can no longer sustain its metabolic activity. The best example is a grain of cereal, which will not spoil for thousands of years if it is stored correctly. Grains found in Egyptian tombs can still germinate today if they are planted in good soil. They still contain enzymes and other vital ingredients needed for our own growth and health. A cereal grain is composed of the following parts: the husk, the flower and the seed. The smallest part is the seed, which guarantees the propagation of the cereal species. Although its weight is only 10 per cent of the entire grain, the seed nevertheless contains all the enzymes and other nutrients. However, because of all these enzymes, the seed tastes a little bitter and, for commercial reasons, this is a disadvantage. It also becomes rancid very quickly and so not only the husk, but also the seed, is discarded during the process of grinding. The husk and the seed are then sold as high-quality animal feed. What is left is the flower, which contains only calories and hardly any essential nutrients. As in the case of most other industrialised food, 'living' food has been turned into a 'dead' product and the animals get the better deal.

When, in the year 1900, the well-known Swiss physician Max Bircher-Benner spoke to an audience of physicians in Zurich, Switzerland, nobody seemed to understand quite what he meant when he talked about the dynamic healing power of raw food and vegetables. They were not able to understand that raw vegetables contain very special nutrients that no longer exist when the vegetable is cooked. The general comment after his lecture was that 'Dr Bircher-Benner had gone beyond the borders of science'. But as he became more and more successful with his special diet, many intelligent physicians became interested in his therapy. In his clinic in Zurich, Dr Bircher-Benner treated not only Swiss patients, but also many patients from the USA, Australia and even Japan with raw vegetables, fruit and his famous breakfast food, Bircher muesli. This is similar to our Granola, and its most important ingredient is a freshly grated apple, which provides the correct nutritional balance in the muesli. Further research has largely confirmed his ideas.

In the year 1949, Dr Hans-Peter Rusch wrote in his work *The Circulation of Living Substances* that in everything alive, there must be tiny 'living units' which 'transfer life' from one being to another. From the rays of the sun we receive our most important source of energy, not only directly, but also indirectly through our food. The well-known physical chemist, Wilhelm Oswald, stated many years ago that 'when we eat plants, we eat energy coming from the sun'. At that time, this was only a theory but today we know that it is true. By electro-magnetic measuring methods, by physical and electro-chemical investigations and by many other methods, we can now prove many facts which were, at the beginning of the 20th century, based only upon the well-thought-out hypotheses of some courageous scientists and physicians.

In order to understand the concept of living food, we must first of all look at the soil. A healthy soil contains many substances which plants need for their growth and development, such as nitrogen, potassium, phosphorus and chalk. In order to absorb all these nutrients from the soil, the plant needs help.

The so-called 'micro-flora' in the soil consists of an army of millions of bacteria, fungi and other micro-organisms which help plants to absorb all these nutrients and to eliminate waste. Alongside this micro-flora there is also the macro-flora whose task is to 'digest' the soil and keep it loose. Earthworms, moles and insects, among others, belong to this macro-flora. This 'living' community in the soil, this micro- and macro-flora, should always be well balanced. Only when this flora is healthy and not interfered with is it possible for the plant, with the help of all these tiny creatures, to absorb their nutrients from the soil, and produce important and essential vital nutrients for human beings and animals.

Plants are able, with the help of a green pigment from their leaves and under the influence of sunlight, to create carbohydrates, fats, proteins and other vital substances. If, with our modern agricultural methods, we destroy the micro- and macro-flora instead of improving the soil, the plants can no longer absorb all the nutrients they need. By using artificial fertilisers, on the one hand the essential requirements of the plants are ignored, and on the other hand, they get far too much of certain substances, such as nitrogen. Thus the soil is destroyed to such a degree that the plants living in it contain only a small fraction of their former nutritious value. Many plants become weak and diseased and are then treated with chemical 'healing remedies', just like human beings. In this way, the micro- and macro-flora are destroyed more and more, until the soil becomes a dead substance.

Similar things happen to people who are continually treated with antibiotics and other chemical substances. In the human body, as well as in the soil, bacteria play a vital part in all processes. Our body contains more bacteria than cells, all of which have their own special functions. Only a very small percentage of these bacteria can be classified as harmful, or even dangerous.

DIFFERENT KINDS OF FAT
We need fat, but not just any kind of fat. Some fat is good for us, but some is bad for our health. The best fats are natural, unsaturated and

polyunsaturated, which we find in natural foods like avocados or nuts and natural oils which have not been treated industrially or changed in any way. However, as soon as these unsaturated fats are heated, they become saturated. Natural unsaturated fats are, because of their biochemical structure, able to combine with natural proteins and thus play an important role in the transportation and utilisation of oxygen in our body. Unsaturated fats are easy to digest, whereas saturated fats can have the same kind of destructive effect on all organic functions as dangerous poisons. They damage the red blood corpuscles, as well as the composition of the blood and, in combination with too much protein, they cause many chronic diseases, such as diabetes, arteriosclerosis, cirrhosis of the liver and thrombosis.

Because of our polluted environment, we find, mainly in animal fat, highly poisonous fat-soluble chemicals such as insecticides, herbicides, detergents, etc. These harmful animal fats, as well as synthetic fats, impair oxygen utilisation and respiratory processes, which are extremely important for a healthy metabolism.

Amongst the animal fats, I can only recommend butter, as almost all kinds of margarine are lifeless industrial products and hardly ever contain healthy unsaturated fats. Although butter contains some saturated fats, it also contains many substances which are absolutely vital to our health. If, once in a while, you eat meat that contains some fat, it will not kill you. However, do not make a habit of it. On the other hand, an avocado pear contains the right kind of fat, and you certainly will not gain any weight when you eat half an avocado from time to time – but please, with some lemon juice and not with mayonnaise.

Natural, unsaturated fats lower the cholesterol content in the blood, prevent blood clotting and lower the blood pressure. They help against infections, prevent thrombosis and liver damage, and also have a soothing effect on the nervous system. Nervous, hyperactive children should regularly take some unsaturated oil, about two or three teaspoonfuls daily. In health shops you will find good unsaturated oils, which you should always keep in the refrigerator, as otherwise they soon become rancid. Vitamin C, magnesium, vitamin B and, above all, zinc, will help children to digest and utilise healthy, unsaturated fat.

FOOD ADDITIVES

Until about 100–150 years ago, only natural means of preserving food were known. Food was dried in the sun, in the air or at the fireplace, or was preserved by the use of sugar, salty or sour liquids, oil or starches. Later, preservation was achieved through heat and eventually by using very low temperatures or ice.

I still remember my grandmother's pantry, where she kept all her homemade jellies, her eggs, sausages, potatoes and uncountable other foods. Her pantry was always full of surprises and she often conjured up delicacies she had been keeping in there for months.

When food has not been changed by mechanical or chemical methods, freezing or drying are still the best and healthiest ways of preserving it. However, as soon as fresh, natural food has been processed and adulterated by industrial manipulation in order to become non-perishable, it becomes a low quality food which has lost all, or at least a great part, of its vital ingredients. Although some of these products still contain proteins, carbohydrates and fats, these have generally been changed to such an extent that they become worthless, harmful or even dangerous for our health when we eat them regularly.

The preserving of food has become a very important commercial factor. About 80 per cent of all food in supermarkets today has been treated in many different ways in order to increase its shelf life or improve its appearance. When a natural product is processed, it loses its attractive appearance, taste and smell. Today this is no longer a problem. The chemical industry offers many substances that will enhance the taste and smell of anything and can change even the most appalling-looking and smelling food into a gourmet dream which says, 'Buy me!' In 1950, about 700 such additives were already officially permitted for use. Today there are over 4,000 additives available and they all contain hardly any natural ingredients.

It is such a pity that our organism does not produce any digestive juices that could digest additives! Many of the additives that are used for food preserving can paralyse or even kill the bacteria which happen to be present in the food. People do not seem to realise that bacteria and human cells are very similar, both of them having their own metabolism, and both are highly sensitive to strong toxins. We may therefore assume that such additives, when taken into our body, could have a similar effect on human cells as they have on bacteria. However, nobody seems to worry about this and, as long as there is no proof beyond doubt that some of these additives are really dangerous for our health, the authorities will do nothing about them and their use will not be restricted.

Every year, more people suffer from incurable diseases whose causes are still unknown, and nobody has yet been able to prove that these have any relation to certain toxic substances which have been accumulating in the body, often for a great number of years. Many people, especially those responsible for the prosperity of industrial enterprise, always point out that the extremely small quantities of additives used are completely harmless. However, there is plenty of proof, for example when using homoeopathic remedies or vaccines, that the human organism can react strongly to infinitely small quantities of toxic or non-toxic substances. Even Catherine de Medici killed her enemies using only the smallest amount of poison!

The human body has not been equipped with anything which could be used to detoxify the ever-growing quantity of foreign substances we consume day by day. Some of those cannot be excreted and remain somewhere in the body, where they start to accumulate. These substances hinder metabolism as well as many other functions of the organism, and very little is yet known about what might happen when different toxins come into contact with each other, producing dangerous cross-reactions. Although in medicine we have known about these problems for many decades, the food industry completely ignores the fact that such reactions could be detrimental to our health: so many autistic children are the victims of too much gluten, sugar, additives, cheese, and especially artificially coloured sweets.

ADDICTIVE AND UNSUITABLE DRINKS
Many people nowadays like to drink coffee, black tea, hot chocolate, soft drinks, alcoholic drinks, or milk (which as we have seen is often quite indigestible) instead of water. Coffee and other drinks containing caffeine stimulate the taste buds in the mouth. They also stimulate the digestive juices in the stomach, increase the heartbeat

and the functions of the brain, help temporarily against migraine headache, and stimulate urine production and bowel movement.

These reactions may last only a few minutes, or sometimes several hours. Then the counter-reaction starts. The coffee drinker gets more and more nervous and sometimes shaky, melancholic or depressive. Habitual coffee drinking can be the cause of serious or chronic migraines. The coffee drinker tends to sip his or her favourite beverage very often, and some people drink up to eight cups of coffee or more per day. In the long run, caffeine is a nerve poison; cola drinks are often the cause of the highly strung state of some children. Sleeplessness and depression are only some of the problems from which caffeine drinkers suffer.

Those who make a habit of drinking alcohol may be creating severe health problems for themselves. Since the First World War, the consumption of coffee and sweet drinks has increased tenfold and the number of alcoholics is frightening. Because coffee and alcohol stimulate kidney function and water elimination from the reserves of the body, these drinks can really dehydrate the body.

Most children like chocolate milk. Prof. Mommsen, a well-known German paediatrician, wrote on the subject: 'Chocolate drinks often contain between 60 – 70 per cent of sugar and for this reason should be rejected.' These drinks also contain quite indigestible cacao, caffeine and saturated fats.

Chocolate can provoke serious allergies, and the degree of saturation is so high that when children eat or drink chocolate, they often lose their natural appetite. It is a big problem that these drinks do not contain the natural complementary substances which enable chocolate milk to be properly digested. (The same applies to any kind of chocolate, which is a vitamin and mineral robber.) However, these drinks sell very well and are hugely popular. Business always comes before health, and may even be legally protected. When they are thirsty most children ask for sweet drinks. Although at first some of these drinks are thirst-quenching, after a short time the child again becomes thirsty because of the sugar content in them. Of course, this is the intention of the manufacturer.

Often when I inform mothers about how bad these soft drinks are for their children, they tell me that their kids are already addicted to the stuff and they do not know how to get them out of this habit. I know this is a big problem. However, much depends on the age of the child in question. As soon as children are big enough to be able to listen to reason – perhaps from the time they are six or seven years old – you can try to explain what kind of harm these drinks do to the body. Do this in a simple and logical way. Never forbid something without a logical explanation – that would be an insult to the intelligence of the child. Tell sporty children that their muscles will grow weak from eating sweets and drinking soft drinks and that they will not be good at sports any more. Tell image-conscious teenagers how ugly they will become when their skin is covered with acne and point out other teenagers who have this problem. Most children will listen. When speaking in schools, I discovered that children are often wiser and more open-minded than their parents and grandparents. It's up to you to explain it in the right way. You will also have to convince the rest of your family of what you are saying, and this might be even harder. Try to become knowledgeable on the subject.

I know how difficult it is for children as they do like fizzy drinks and fruit squash. I think, however, that as well as natural fruit juices (which are allowed), fresh water is very important. Be very careful with sugary, fizzy lemonades as this might be detrimental to the child. Look at the foods which are alive and which will help hyperactive or autistic children to cope with their problems. It will be worth it, especially when living with an autistic child, as in that case one would do anything one could to help.

It is important that the subject of allergies and the importance of healthy, natural food is understood, and this should be applied not only to mothers and children, but also to fathers. Your reward will be a healthy family.

TEN

The Great Vaccination Dilemma

'The microbe is nothing, the terrain is everything.'
Louis Pasteur

Life can be complicated, especially where children are concerned. For new parents, there are many lifestyle adjustments to make when a baby comes home. Simply getting to grips with your child's routine and needs takes some time, not to mention regaining your own health after nine months of pregnancy and the rigours of childbirth! Then, eight weeks later, just as the dust is settling, comes a major decision – do you follow the recognised path and agree to a full set of childhood vaccinations, select just a few or avoid them altogether? There can be no easy answer to this dilemma, which may be a good thing in the long run since it forces a judgement to be made on the basis of an informed decision, which, in turn, can only be made once both sides of the argument are heard.

In this chapter, I will present some ideas and concepts that may, on first inspection, appear to offer a negative perspective on the immunisation process, but this is not my aim. I wish to deliver a biological argument that challenges the wholesale immunisation of our infant population in favour of improving and optimising a child's natural ecology, or terrain as Louis Pasteur aptly described it. In so doing, it is possible to enhance and optimise your child's overall health and well-being. It would be inappropriate to attempt to show that immunisations 'don't work', since numerous scientific papers clearly show that they do assist in controlling disease epidemics.

Again, it is not my aim to disprove the effectiveness of a given immunisation programme, but I do want to raise the suggestion that a fully immunised child population may not be as healthy as we once thought or expected it should be. I think it is important to remember that immunisations are no guarantee of immunity against disease, and there is growing concern expressed by many parents and some holistically orientated health professionals that, in trying to protect our children, we could be priming their bodies for health problems later in life.

Only today I spoke to a mother whose three-year-old daughter was confirmed as suffering from whooping cough, despite being fully immunised against the disease. When this point was raised, her doctor told her that the whooping cough vaccine was only about 70 per cent effective and that she may have had a much worse case if she had not been immunised. The child's mother commented that her daughter had been fine before she was vaccinated and only developed the problem ten days after her boosters. This was dismissed as pure coincidence. Keeping in mind that the little girl was already an asthma sufferer (starting coincidentally just after her first set of jabs when she was ten weeks of age), one could jump to conclusions and start pointing an accusing finger at the immunisation process. However, what evidence, if any, exists to support such an indictment?

The fact is that this accusation borrows considerable support from observations made in a paper published in the medical journal *The Lancet* in 1996.[3] In the June issue, a group of scientists studying the spread of disease, introduced their feature by stating that 'the rise in allergic disease among children in the UK over the past 30 years remains unexplained'. This comment, taken in isolation, in no way points an accusing finger at immunisations, but the authors do go on to refine their theory by stating that 'one hypothesis is that infections in early childhood prevent allergic sensitisation (i.e. the development of an allergic state), and that successive generations of children have lost this protection as their exposure to infectious disease early in life has declined'. The authors do not recommend getting ill just to prevent allergies in later life, but it does underpin an important fundamental aspect of our immune response – that contracting infections is an important and powerful driving force behind developing a strong and effective immune response that lasts a lifetime. Following this line of thinking, it is interesting to note that just as the rates of measles and whooping cough infections have fallen 100-fold over the past 50 years, the prevalence of allergy and related diseases has sharply risen over the past 30 years. To add some numbers to this discussion, an audit from the National Asthma Campaign (1997/98)[4] showed that one in seven children (aged two to fifteen) in the UK have asthma severe enough to require daily treatment. The latest audit (2001)[5] sadly shows that things are getting worse, with a rise in the estimated prevalence of asthma from 3.4 million in 1999 to 5.1 million adults and children today. However, this could be just the tip of the iceberg! Consider how many children may have mild asthma whose parents wish to avoid steroid-based inhalers, or who have simply slipped through the diagnostic net altogether. These children do not get included in audits since there is no documented record of their illness to analyse.

Some asthma may be considered 'intrinsic' or part of their genetic make-up, but for the majority of sufferers it can be viewed as an illness caused by allergies, normally to dust, milk and other inhaled triggers, such as pollens and animal hair. This allergic reaction is driven by an antibody known as IGE. As immunologist Prof. Graham Rook of University College London Medical School clearly put it, 'give us this day our daily germs', the title of his paper published in the journal *Immunology Today*.[6] Rook's article highlights the key interplay between infections and a healthy immune system. He describes how 'modern vaccinations, fear of germs and obsession with hygiene are depriving the immune system of the information input upon which it is dependent'. Prof. Rook goes on to explain how this alters the fine chemical balance of the body and may be at the heart of our allergy explosion, and suggests that: 'If humans continue to deprive their immune system of the input to which evolution has adapted it, it may be necessary to devise ways of replacing it artificially.' He concludes by making suggestions for developing vaccines, including designing vaccines that do not merely protect from infections, but maintain the correct internal chemical environment which, in turn, encourages the power of our natural immune mechanisms. This modern proposal for health appears to mirror Louis Pasteur's original comment that 'the microbe is nothing, the terrain is everything'.

The history of immunisation is greater and older than Louis Pasteur or even the father of modern vaccination, Edward Jenner. For centuries, druids and other healers have been using the concept of preparing the body for a disease through introducing it to a small dose of that disease. Even the father of homoeopathy, Samuel Hahnemann, was an advocate of vaccination. However, immunisation by injection into the bloodstream is a modern idea. In Jenner's day, cowpox was introduced into the body via a scratch on the skin rather than by direct injection deep in the body and directly into the bloodstream. As for Hahnemann, the use of single remedies taken by mouth formed the cornerstone of his vaccination methods.

The vaccination methods of Jenner and Hahnemann, and those of modern medicine, generate two very different immune reactions. These may not necessarily be different in process, but are quite different in intensity. A simple scratch with an infected knife or needle, such as that used by Jenner, or a single homoeopathically prepared remedy, allowed the infective agent a slow passage into the body, giving the immune mechanisms time to mount a reaction. There was not the overwhelming 'all or nothing' response that typically follows immunisation by injection.

By introducing the vaccine by injection, a massive amount of a limited variety of antibodies are produced. So many, in fact, that the immune system's capacity to mount an effective response against other non-vaccinated illnesses can become compromised. This is the reason why doctors don't advise you to vaccinate your child if he or she has a cold or is otherwise unwell. The stress placed on the immune system by the vaccination process is so great that a drop in its ability to deal with opportunistic infection is produced. This effect is often recognised by parents who repeatedly take their child to the doctor with recurrent infections of the ears, nose and chest. It seems from talking to parents that these problems often start at about nine or ten weeks of age, soon after the first round of vaccinations. Could this be pure coincidence, or is there a connection between immune 'overload' and increased susceptibility to chronic minor infections? Admittedly, children are prone to these problems since they tend to pick up every bug going, but it appears that many more children are developing long-term congestive ear problems and allergic conditions such as asthma, eczema and food allergies.

The current UK vaccination programme[7] is introduced at eight weeks of age with a combination of four viruses (diphtheria, tetanus and pertussis [whooping cough], or DTP, along with Hib) in one injection, one virus (polio) in a single oral dose and another virus (meningitis C) in another single injection. Is it any wonder that some babies suffer immediate reactions? Even though one may acknowledge that immunisation can play a part in controlling disease epidemics, do we need to pump six different agents into eight-week-old babies, five of which are injected directly into the body along with their additives, such as aluminium salts, formaldehyde and egg proteins, to mention but a few? Why, for example, does an eight-week-old baby need a tetanus shot when they are unlikely to play outside, let alone suffer a deep enough wound to contract tetanus infection? According to a feature in the *British Medical Journal*,[8] immunisation for tetanus does not rule out contracting tetanus. In a few cases, it has been clearly shown that, despite adequate vaccine cover, tetanus can still occur!

However, until a few years ago, there was no decision to make. We all routinely made an appointment with the doctor and had our children vaccinated against the common childhood diseases. Despite this, concerns have risen over the past few years regarding the potentially harmful long-term effects of giving children multiple vaccinations despite repeated reassurances from the Department of Health. These worries have been brought to the fore following the published results from the Royal Free Hospital into the connection between the MMR (mumps, measles and rubella) vaccination, autism and inflammatory bowel disease. The research was published in the medical journal *The Lancet*[9] and concluded that the onset of bowel inflammation and autistic behaviour was, in the majority of cases, closely linked to the administration of the MMR vaccination. The doctors responsible for the study described in their report how children with a history of normal growth and development rapidly lost acquired skills such as language, as they started to display classic autistic behavioural problems in addition to gut upsets, such as diarrhoea, pain, food intolerance and bloating. In most cases, the onset of symptoms followed MMR vaccination!

News of this discovery made the headlines and received considerable media attention with the predictable knee-jerk response from the medical profession. Sadly, the study, and the scientists and doctors who conducted it, were somewhat discredited by their peers. However, a couple of years later, similar reports of an unexplained rise in developmental abnormalities appeared from America. In 1999, Dr Bernard Rimland, founder of the Autism Research Institute in San Diego,[10] claimed that 'the rates are rising because of the overuse of vaccines'.[11] Dr Rimland's data suggests cases of autism have trebled in America; in California they have nearly quadrupled! Understandably, a spokesman for Merck & Co, which makes the MMR vaccine, said, 'There is absolutely nothing in medical or scientific literature that would suggest a link between vaccinations and autism.' I am sure we have not heard the end of this tale.

From a parent's point of view, the wealth of information currently available from books, journals and the Internet has made the decision to vaccinate or not a nightmare. The pressure to vaccinate is great. 'Be wise and immunise' is the advice given by health visitors and doctors, and well-meaning family and friends often make you feel compelled to follow the established convention. However, there is an ever-mounting body of evidence that offers compelling reasons not to vaccinate, or at least to vaccinate using a select few single vaccines. In order, however, to make an informed decision, parents must understand the potential outcomes from both scenarios. Several parent support groups have appeared, the best connected of which is the JABS organisation.[12] However, depending on who has written the information, you may receive a very extreme point of view for or against vaccination. Either way, there are some facts that cannot be argued, some of which highlight fundamental weaknesses in the vaccination process itself.

By definition, vaccinations introduce into the body the very agents that the body is designed to keep out or fight: viruses. The concept is that, following a vaccination, a small dose of inactivated virus stimulates the body to make antibodies that will recognise the 'real thing' should the body ever come across it again. In other words, the body is primed and ready to fight common childhood infections if an outbreak occurs. This theory sounds great, but don't forget there is no such thing as a free lunch! It is difficult to imagine when, in nature, a young animal would ever contract six illnesses at once, yet we are happy to give our babies two injections and one oral dose, all of which are powerful enough to stimulate a massive antibody reaction in one go, and expect a beneficial response.

Table 2: Current Department of Health guidelines regarding immunisation (2001)

Vaccinations given during the first year of life
(18 exposures to viral vaccines)

Age	Vaccines
At 8 weeks	DTP (triple combination + Hib), meningitis C (single injection), polio (by mouth)
At 12 weeks	DTP (triple combination + Hib), meningitis C (single injection), polio (by mouth)
At 16 weeks	DTP (triple combination + Hib), meningitis C (single injection), polio (by mouth)

Vaccinations given during the second year of life
(3 exposures to viral vaccines)

Age	Vaccine
At 15 months	MMR (triple combination)

Booster vaccinations given before starting school
(7 exposures to viral vaccines)

Age	Vaccine
At 3–4 years	DTP (triple combination + Hib), polio (by mouth), MMR (triple combination)
At 10–14 years	BCG (tuberculosis)
At 13–18 years	Diphtheria, tetanus and polio

Studies into Gulf War syndrome may be an unlikely place to uncover facts about the effects of childhood vaccinations on the immune system, but this has opened up new areas of research, suggesting that individual vaccines may themselves not be a problem, but combining them may be.

The sufferers of Gulf War syndrome exhibited many signs that indicated an immune-based problem. After many years of fighting, the Ministry of Defence admitted that, against the advice from its own research centre at Porten Down, it gave potent and potentially dangerous combinations of vaccines to the troops prior to leaving for the Gulf. The findings were published in the scientific journal *Nature*.[13] The importance of this was highlighted in another of Prof. Rook's articles,[14] discussing the implications of vaccine combinations on the chemistry of the immune system. Prof. Rook suggests that certain vaccine combinations push the body's chemistry into an inflammatory and pro-allergic state. To use an unavoidable medical term, the body is pushed into a 'Th2 cytokine shift'. A cytokine is simply a chemical that acts on the body's cells to exert an effect or change. A Th2 cytokine represents a specific type of cytokine that tends to promote inflammation, allergy and the production of large amounts of the key antibody IgE. People who have a predominantly Th2 cytokine profile normally display all kinds of chronic allergic symptoms – asthma, eczema and the like. After much research, it was discovered that the pertussis (whooping cough) part of the DTP vaccine that could prove troublesome for childhood immunisations was also shown to be the culprit in Gulf War syndrome: pertussis was combined with the anthrax vaccine in order to make the anthrax vaccine work quicker. The resultant cocktail became the focus of interest for those scientists investigating Gulf War syndrome victims.

As far as we can see, despite much reassurance from the conventional health authorities, there is much controversy and research interest in vaccine combinations and their effect on the immune system. In addition to this, there is a definite rise in immune-based illness such as asthma, eczema, food and contact allergies, nasal and ear infections/congestion and inflammatory bowel disease. Admittedly, apart from asthma and some severe cases of inflammatory bowel disease, these problems may not be life-threatening, but the fact exists that something is perverting the healthy direction of many children's immune systems.

What, if any, alternatives exist to the conventional immunisation programme? If you talk to homoeopaths, you will get very different stories depending on their background. Those homoeopaths who belong to the Faculty of Homoeopaths will be very pro-immunisation since they are medically qualified homoeopaths. To support their stance, they will quote the fact that Hahnemann was also an advocate of immunisation and they are, in fact, following in the steps of his teachings. What they don't mention is the fact that Hahnemann used single homoeopathic vaccine remedies administered by mouth and did not use the multiple cocktails of injected vaccines, as used today. Those homoeopaths who belong to the Society of Homoeopaths, for example, are not medically qualified homoeopaths, they are homoeopathically qualified homoeopaths and stand firmly behind the idea of avoiding vaccinations where possible. They may recommend a programme somewhat like that described below.

Table 3: Homoeopathic Alternatives

Vaccine	How to Take
Diphtheria	*Diphtherinum 30* (nosode): 1 dose weekly for 1 month during times of suspected epidemic or risk from infection.
Measles	*Morbillinum 30* (nosode): 1 dose weekly for 1 month during times of suspected epidemic or risk from infection.
Mumps	*Parotidinum 30* (nosode): 1 dose weekly for 1 month during times of suspected epidemic or risk from infection.
Polio	*Poliomyelitis 30* (nosode): 1 dose weekly for 1 month during times of suspected epidemic or risk from infection.
Rubella	*Rubella 30* (nosode): 1 dose weekly for 1 month during times of suspected epidemic or risk from infection. Can also be taken by pregnant women who have come into contact with the disease.

| Tetanus | *Clostridium tetani 30* (nosode): 1 dose weekly for 1 month during times of suspected epidemic or risk from infection. |
| Whooping cough | *Pertussin 30* (nosode): 1 dose weekly for 1 month during times of suspected epidemic or risk from infection. |

* *The advice of a professional homoeopath is always recommended, but these special remedies are available by mail order from Ainsworth's Homoeopathic Pharmacy, 0207 935 5330.*

The immunisation process appears to behave rather like a double-edged sword. There is a trade-off between the prevention of diseases that are largely non-fatal for an increased susceptibility to chronic minor infections and allergic-based health problems. The importance of diet, nutritional quality of food and hygiene cannot be over-estimated in determining disease outcome. Most of the tragic outcomes from childhood illness occur in those children who were poorly nourished, in poor general health and often living in crowded unhygienic surroundings. This point of view was upheld by Dr Bernard Dixon of the World Health Organisation, who stated that 'the most valuable immunisation is good nutrition'.

Diet and nutrition, therefore, play a key role in the overall health of children, especially in the formative years when illness is commonplace.

The importance of breast-feeding cannot be overstated. The mother's antibody protection comes across in the breast milk, providing the baby with passive immunity against all the diseases that the mother has contracted during her life. When breast-feeding stops, the baby's antibody levels drop after a few months. Many naturopaths recommend drinking cabbage juice during breast-feeding. This can stimulate your body to produce more protective antibodies. However, some babies may be sensitive to chemicals in cabbages that come across in the maternal milk, giving them wind and colic.

From a purely nutritional point of view, during the weaning time try to introduce your child to a variety of foods including those with high levels of vitamins A, C and E and the minerals zinc and selenium. These specific nutrients are known to boost the natural immune function and stimulate white blood cell function.

Good immune-boosting foods to feed infants when weaning are: carrots, boiled and mashed (high in carotenoids, which are made into vitamin A by the body); mango, steamed and mashed (high in vitamin C); avocado, mashed (good source of vitamin E); lamb, cooked very well and mixed with sweet potato (good supply of zinc and carotenoids) and natural bio-yoghurt, which contains live cultures that can boost the body's gut population of friendly bacteria which, in turn, boosts the immune cell population.

In conclusion, the choice is yours. I hope that this chapter has not been the deciding factor in your choice to vaccinate or not, but will rather form one source of information, presenting every side of the argument, for you to mull over. In this age of high-tech medicine, the belief that mass vaccination is the best way to protect the health of the nation needs to be studied further. We are well aware that tinkering with nature can have some unpleasant repercussions, such as antibiotic-resistant infections and the increasing incidence of breast cancers associated with the long-term use of oestrogen-only hormone replacement therapy. Maybe some day we will be viewing multiple vaccinations and their effects on the immune system in a similar way.

ELEVEN

A–Z of Childhood Illnesses

What are childhood illnesses? Very often these are infectious diseases caused by viruses or bacteria. They usually run like other infectious diseases. The virus develops into a bacteria, often without any cause for alarm. The incubation time can take a few days or possibly even a few weeks and, when it develops, the child can become very ill. The only comfort is that children get these diseases only once; the immune system will usually stop them getting the disease a second time.

What can one do about them? Basically, for these particular childhood diseases there is no cure. You can, however, help by easing the child's discomfort, so that the temperature lowers, the pain or itch is relieved and the breathing becomes easier. Luckily, most childhood diseases are not worrying. If medical guidance during the attacks is helpful, a lot can be done. There are, of course, a few illnesses that are very dangerous, such as whooping cough or polio. Those particular problems can mostly be prevented by vaccination.

Is there any form of protection? As I stated in the last chapter, vaccination against really life-threatening childhood diseases is an option. However, as I have already said, it is very important to handle vaccination and immunisation with care.

Can childhood diseases affect adults? Usually not. Most adults have already had illnesses such as measles, chickenpox and scarlet fever. It is always very important to take proper action if these illnesses are contracted by adults, however.

There are all kinds of home remedies that one can take, and in my book *Questions and Answers on Family Health*, I have given examples of many. It is important that childhood illnesses are properly treated. Today, we are a nation of chronic invalids because we suppress diseases through medication that removes the symptoms. We often treat childhood diseases by trying to control fevers, or by giving antibiotics too quickly. But what is in the body has to come out, and I agree with the naturopathic principle that you have to sweat to eliminate toxins. Don't try to control things too quickly. When the temperature rises, it is probably time to take some action with cold-water compresses. However, keep the child in bed to 'really sweat it out', as the old people used to say in Holland.

Give the child fruit or vegetable juices, such as beetroot juice, which is very good for childhood diseases because it works as a wonderful antioxidant. Administer some natural antibiotics, such as Echinaforce, or use cough mixture (when there is a lot of coughing) like Sure Cure. Whatever you do, take proper advice and allow these childhood diseases to work their way out of the system as much as possible. There is so much that one can do to help.

Over the years that I have worked in this field, I have seen many despairing parents whose child could not sleep because of colic, and kept the parents awake into the bargain. This is easily solved: simply put a slice of onion into a cup of hot water, leave it to steep until the water is lukewarm and then give the child a teaspoonful. This relieves the colic very quickly. With all of the allergies, there are many desensitisers that can help the child. When a child cannot sleep, it is very easy to relax the body by giving a little *Valerian hops*.

There are hundreds of ways to treat childhood illnesses. In this A–Z I will give some advice on quick and easy treatments that I have used successfully over the 45 years I have been in practice. There are many books on the subject of how to treat childhood diseases, so this is only a very short summary. It is intended for quick and easy reference when first aid is required.

With both mother and child, it is often important to look at the little things and nip them in the bud to make sure that minor ailments do not develop into more serious conditions. The more naturally you can do this, the better. Nature is a tremendous treasure of remedies and, especially for children, these are always of the greatest help. *Questions and Answers on Family Health* gives more detailed explanations of the conditions that often occur and need immediate action.

A

ABDOMINAL PAIN: When the child has abdominal discomfort or swelling, place your left hand on the tummy (right under the naval) and put your right hand over this. Breathe in deeply into your own tummy and out of the mouth (matching your breath to that of the baby). This will very often offer relief. If the abdominal swelling doesn't go away, you can give the child two drops of *Centaurium* in a little water and this will be of tremendous help.

ADENOIDS: Be careful about adenoids and always consult your doctor. If as the child gets older adenoids are still a problem, administer five drops of *Marum verum* twice a day. Be careful about milk and cheese, as they may aggravate the problem, but encourage the child to eat some honey.

ALLERGIES: Identify the allergy first. There are many ways one can test for allergies nowadays. When you start to omit certain foods, make sure that the child doesn't become deficient in any nutrients, and take some proper advice. The child can take half a tablet of ALR formula twice a day, which is a good desensitiser.

ASTHMA: Always make sure that your GP is aware of the problem and recognises what kind of asthma the child has. This is very important, in order to ensure that the child can be properly treated. With asthma, you often have to be careful about the intake of milk and cheese. There are some very good simple remedies that can be of help, such as Ivy-Thyme Complex (taken as described on the bottle) and Sure Cure, but make sure that you seek professional advice.

B

BEDWETTING: Treatment of bedwetting is different depending on whether the child is a boy or a girl. With boys, I usually advise that the child takes ten drops of *Galeopsis* (which is an excellent remedy) twice a day; you can also rub St John's Wort oil all over the bladder area before the child goes to sleep. Don't let the child drink after 5 p.m. Another herbal remedy, *Uva-Ursi*, is also beneficial. With girls, use *Pulsatilla* (twice a day, five drops) instead, along with the St John's Wort oil treatment. These remedies are usually of great help, but if they do not work acupuncture or laser treatment will be of great assistance.

BITES: Wasp, bee or other insect bites or stings, and even dog bites, can be treated successfully with the homoeopathic remedy *Ledum Pal* 30c.

BROKEN BONES: When the child breaks a bone, you should administer some *Urticalcin* (two tablets twice a day) or *Silica* (one tablet twice a day), to aid quick recovery after the bone has been set by the hospital.

BRONCHITIS: Bronchitis can usually be relieved by a good diet. Avoid any dairy products from cows, take extra honey and use Echinaforce and the remedy Ivy-Thyme Complex with perhaps some Sure Cure. This will help ensure that things clear up very quickly.

BRUISES: Bruises can be quickly treated with the homeopathic remedy *Arnica*. *Arnica* 30c is always of great help, and one can also use *Arnica* ointment externally. A remedy that I find treats bruises well is *Ung Em*. This may be obtained from the herbalists Abbots of Leigh.

BURNS: It is very important that the cleansing and dressing of burns is taken care of properly. St John's Wort oil or the homoeopathic remedy *Cantharis* are both good. It is also very important that the child gets some help to recover from the shock of the burns. You should administer some Emergency Essence.

C

CATARRH: Catarrh conditions are very often caused by wrong dietary management. I usually suggest cutting milk and cheese out of the diet. To ease the catarrh, Echinaforce and the remedy Sure Cure will be of great benefit.

CHEST INFECTIONS: Consult your doctor if your child has a chest infection. Usually chest infections of any kind will be helped by the use of Echinaforce and five drops of *Lachesis* D12 taken twice a day will be of very great help.

CHICKENPOX: To help the child get over chickenpox as quickly as possible, the homoeopathic remedy *Rhus tox* (taken twice a day, five drops) is always very useful.

CHILBLAINS: These can be relieved with *Pulsatilla* and *Rhus tox*, and by the excellent ointment Dalet balm, which can help this condition greatly.

COLD SORES: After the age of one, a child may take one capsule of *Anduvite,* which would be of very great help.

COLDS: Can be treated by some extra Echinaforce. Another excellent remedy is half a glass of hot water with a teaspoonful of honey, the juice of half a lemon and some drops of Echinaforce, depending on the age of the child. This will help to get the cold out of the system.

COLIC: Colic is one of the biggest health problems in childhood. I usually advise on giving the child the onion remedy described above: add a slice of onion to a glass of hot water, leave to cool until lukewarm and give the child a teaspoonful. Some fennel water or *Centaurium* may also be very helpful.

CONCUSSION: Always use *Arnica* and Emergency Essence.

CONJUNCTIVITIS: *Euphrasia* is of great help (five drops twice a day), but *Arnica* will also give a lot of good results for any eye problem.

CONSTIPATION: A common problem. Please ensure that the child does not have sores and that the rectal area is not cracked. Provide plenty of exercise, fluids and fruit juice. You should also put a few grains of Linoforce (which is chocolate-coated) over the child's food.

CONVULSIONS: Always speak to your doctor if your child has a convulsion. After taking the doctor's advice, you can also give one tablet of *Kelpasan*, which will be of very great help.

COUGHS: Any kind of cough should not be ignored. It is an alarm bell that something is not right. With most coughs, Sure Cure is a tremendous help. If it is deep in the chest, I usually advise SP Chest, and sucking some *Santasapina* bon-bons is also good.

CRADLE CAP: St John's Wort oil or diluted cider vinegar, rubbed into the scalp, is usually of great assistance.

CROUP: Although not very common nowadays, it is important if there is croup to use the remedy *Mercurius heel*, one tablet twice a day. Also, *Aconite* is often effective.

CUTS: St John's Wort oil has a healing effect with cuts, or use *Ung A* ointment from Abbots of Leigh.

D

DERMATITIS: You should take the child to see your GP straight away. Use *Ung E* from Abbots of Leigh.

DIARRHOEA: Never ignore diarrhoea. Use Tormentil Complex (twice a day, five drops), and Bowel Essence is also great.

DIPHTHERIA: While the child is being treated by the doctor, you can give complementary help with Echinaforce.

DYSLEXIA: This needs professional guidance, but the homoeopathic remedy *Cerebium* is of complementary assistance.

E

EARACHE: Earache should be very carefully handled. A good remedy is *Plantago* (five drops twice a day). Also, put five drops of *Plantago* on a piece of cotton wool, and place this deeply in the ear at bedtime. This often solves the problem. The homoeopathic remedy *Tuberculinum* (IM potency) can also be used. I often advise patients with earache to drink chamomile tea.

ECZEMA: There are many different types of eczema, but with the three main ones it is usually quite helpful to keep off dairy foods. Often infantile eczema and asthma are caused by taking a child off breast milk and putting it on cows' milk, so watch this very carefully. Violaforce, a herbal remedy, is very helpful for eczema. Get some professional advice from a homeopath as there are lots of remedies which are very effective. *Ung E* ointment is excellent.

EYE INFECTIONS: Always get professional advice for any problem to do with the delicate eye area. You could help by putting a little Epsom salts in a cup of hot water and when it is lukewarm, giving the eyes a wash.

F

FEVER: As my grandmother used to say, 'Give me a fever and I will treat all ills.' A very good way to treat all fevers and get the illness out the system is to take some cold or hot water packs, as described in my book *Water – Healer or Poison?* Echinaforce is also very helpful.

FRACTURES: To help heal fractures, *Arnica*, Emergency Essence and *Urticalcin* are very effective.

G

GASTROENTERITIS: This condition requires advice from your health visitor and should be treated by your doctor. Sometimes a few drops of *Centaurium* may be beneficial.

GERMAN MEASLES: Another infectious disease that needs very careful handling and consultation with your doctor. Give the child some Echinaforce.

GLUE EAR: The remedy *Plantago* may be used to treat this. Five drops should be taken internally twice a day, and five drops on a piece of cotton wool placed in the ear overnight will be of help.

GROWING PAINS: A common problem. *Arnica* will help, and also Emergency Essence.

H

HAYFEVER: Take five drops of *Pollinosan luffa* complex twice a day. Limit milk, cheese and kitchen salt, and include honey in the diet.

HEADACHES: These are often the first indication that something else is wrong in the body. Keep a close eye on the child's health and investigate further.

HEAD LICE: Wash the child's hair with tea tree shampoo and put cider vinegar in the water for the last rinse.

HEPATITIS: Eating artichoke as a vegetable and adding it to soup is of tremendous help but, of course, the guidance of the doctor or health visitor will be necessary.

I

IMPETIGO: Impetigo can be helped with Violaforce (ten drops before meals twice a day) and zinc.

INFLUENZA: Five drops of Influaforce twice a day.

J

JAUNDICE: I have found Milk Thistle Complex to be very beneficial for jaundice. Taken twice a day, five drops is enough. Be very careful with the child's diet.

L

LARYNGITIS: This can be treated with the remedy *Echtrosept*. Five to ten drops should be taken twice a day. Give the child some chamomile tea and use Sure Cure.

M

MEASLES: Consult your doctor if your child develops measles. It is very important to flush measles out of the system as soon as possible. The child must be kept in bed. Use *Rhus tox* and Echinaforce.

MOUTH INFECTIONS: Can be very often cleared with one teaspoon of Molkosan diluted in a cup of water and used as a mouthwash.

MUMPS: Yet another problem that can have far-reaching effects, so always consult your doctor, because if mumps is not properly treated it can affect a man's fertility in later life. I have often seen this when miasmas are left from a former inflammation, virus or infection. With mumps, it is important to use the homoeopathic remedy *Mercurius heel.* One tablet taken twice a day will be of very great help. I must stress that with some cases of infertility, when I have prescribed homoeopathic remedies such as *Belladonna, Chamomilla* and *Mercurius sol* 3X, I have had very good results in clearing the problem, helping couples who couldn't previously have children.

N

NAPPY RASH: *Ung Em* ointment from Abbots of Leigh is of very great help. Use this night and morning.

NOSEBLEEDS: It can be problematic when nosebleeds don't stop. Before any surgical help is required, try an old-fashioned remedy – put a little fresh chicken meat into the nostril to stop bleeding. Also, *Hamamelis virginica* (two or three drops twice a day) can be used, and this is often very effective.

O

OBESITY: This can, of course, be a problem in children. One or two tablets of *Kelpasan,* a safe remedy which helps to speed up the metabolism, can help.

OVERTIRED CHILDREN: With overtired children, it is helpful to use the remedy Vitaforce, a herbal vitamin product which is very tasty. Take one teaspoonful twice a day. Vitamin supplements from Michaels will help.

P

PHARYNGITIS: This can usually be greatly helped with the excellent remedy *Lachesis* taken twice a day (five drops).

PRICKLY HEAT: Solidago Complex taken twice a day (five drops) will be a great help.

R

RASH: Usually a rash will be relieved by Evening Primrose oil or Solidago Complex taken twice a day (five drops).

RINGWORM: Take five drops of the remedy *Harpagophytum* (Devil's claw) twice a day, and also Evening Primrose oil.

RUBELLA: *Rubella nosode* is effective in treating this ailment.

S

SCARLET FEVER: This is a problem which must be professionally diagnosed and treated. Five drops of Influaforce twice a day should also help.

SHOCK: Never ignore shock or trauma. Use Emergency Essence or *Arnica.*

SICKNESS: This can usually be relieved by taking five drops of *Nux vomica* twice a day.

SINUS INFECTIONS: Limit milk and cheese and take some honey. The remedy SNS Formula will be of great help.

SLEEPWALKING: Sleepwalking is usually less common than nightmares in children, but it can lead to some complications. The homoeopathic remedies *Aconite* and *Natrum mur* are often of great help. If the child is very anxious, use *Aconite* 30c. If the sleepwalking begins after the child has had a shock or trauma, give it *Natrum mur* 30c.

SPRAINS: St John's Wort oil is very good for sprains. Apply externally to the affected area.

STOMACH UPSETS: With stomach upsets drink some hot chamomile tea and use the remedy Arabiaforce twice a day (two drops), which usually works very well.

STYES: Taken twice a day, one tablet of *Mercurius heel* will be effective. You could also use the ointment *Ung Em*.

SUNBURN: Be very careful not to allow children to burn, especially babies, but if they do you should immediately get some medical help. To ease sunburn, administer some Emergency Essence internally and St John's Wort oil externally.

SWOLLEN GLANDS: Swollen glands are usually a strong indication that something is wrong, and you should seek medical help. Influaforce is a useful remedy for this ailment and I often prescribe *Lymphomyosot*.

T

TEMPERATURE: When a child has a high temperature, it is always important to consult one's doctor. Echinaforce can help.

TEETHING: With teething, homoeopathic medicine often proves very useful and Nelsons teething granules are very good, or simply use chamomile or *Pulsatilla* . Dabbing a little *Propolis* on the gums is also effective.

THREADWORMS: If nothing else works with threadworms, the

remedy *Papayasan* is usually very effective (one tablet twice a day).

THRUSH: Always make sure that thrush is immediately attended to. Relief will be provided by *Harpagophytum*, but dietary management is also necessary. If it is vaginal thrush, use yoghurt compresses – natural yoghurt is excellent for thrush.

TRAVEL SICKNESS: I find Emergency Essence very good for travel sickness, but the homoeopathic remedy *Cocculus* will make travelling a lot easier for the child who has this problem.

U

ULCERS: Ulcers, both internal and external, are another alarm bell and should be treated. Externally, the ointment Conc E from Abbots helps. Internally, a few drops of *Centaurium* will complement whatever other action is taken.

URINE INFECTIONS: *Echtrosept*, taken twice a day (five drops) before meals, usually clears urine infections. If not, one can use the herbal remedy *Uva-Ursi*.

URTICARIA: Eat fresh fruit and cooked vegetables and, importantly, eat dried fruits. The remedy *Solidago* (five drops twice a day) will be of great help.

V

VAGINAL INFECTIONS: Take five drops of *Echtrosept* twice daily.

VERRUCAS: Dabbing verrucas with *Molkosan* is effective.

VOMITING: Take five drops of *Nux vomica* twice a day.

W

WARTS: Warts are seen as an indication of many problems by homoeopaths. Warts always should be treated and the remedy *Thuja Complex* works well. Five drops taken twice a day will help. Externally, brush on a little *Propolis*.

WAX IN EARS: This can usually be cleared by putting five drops of *Plantago* on a piece of cotton wool and placing it in the ear.

WHOOPING COUGH: This is a nasty infectious problem requiring medical care. However, with whooping cough there are several homoeopathic remedies that can be of help, such as *Veratrum album* or *Pertussin 30* taken once a week during an epidemic, or three doses in one week. The herbal remedies *Belladonna* and *Bryonia* can help, but the problem certainly needs medical attention.

WORMS: With worms, in general it is helpful to give the child plenty of onions and garlic to eat. Be very careful with cheese as this often makes the situation worse. *Papayasan* is very good, and lemon juice also helps.

WOUND HEALING: This is always assisted by Echinaforce, *Arnica* and *Urticalcin*. Depending on the seriousness of the wound, it may be necessary to see your doctor.

X

X-RAYS: When X-rays are absolutely necessary, it is important to take 15 drops of Echinaforce twice a day, as well as vitamin C, to help get rid of any waste material that the X-ray may leave in the body.

TWELVE

Supplements

Being a naturopath at heart, I believe strongly that good nutrition is very important. There are, however, circumstances when supplements should be taken. When problems occur as the child grows up, it is often necessary to introduce certain supplements to his or her diet, which may lack certain vitamins, minerals and trace elements, and these may have to be added to redress the balance. With my own children and grandchildren, I have only recommended supplements when they are absolutely necessary. It is often difficult to know when these are needed and which should be taken, and it is therefore important that professional advice should be sought in the first instance. A combination of good nutrition, exercise and supplements may be needed in certain circumstances.

There might be a problem with the absorption and transportation of nutrition in the process of digestion. Digestion and elimination are interdependent; if nutrients are used properly by the body, there will simultaneously be a continuous and effective process of elimination. Since our energy comes from food, if the child has a deficiency it must be recognised and addressed. The diet must be observed carefully to ensure that the child is getting everything he or she needs nutritionally; if we are not careful, the food we give our children may not be adequate for their needs. Good dietary management is very important.

Until the age of six months, babies will get all the vitamins they need from breast milk or formula milk. As babies grow, the amount of vitamins they need increases. As traditional paediatricians often advise, it is important to make sure that the child gets enough vitamins A and D. When extra vitamins must be added, you can check with a professional who will advise what further action needs to be taken. I can give an example from my experience with one of my own children: when my wife's breast milk was not adequate and formula milk had to be added to my daughter's diet to supplement it, she did need some extra vitamins. These can be given to a baby under professional guidance. In her book *Is This Your Child?* Dr Doris Rapp puts a lot of emphasis on the necessity of vitamins, minerals and trace elements. The research she has done, outlined in her book, clearly demonstrates the need for professional guidance in this matter.

At present nobody can explain how the immune system really works. Immunity, however, is very important for children and the stronger the immunity they build up for the future, the better. When the immune system is low, more help is needed in the form of supplementation. The immune system is the defence mechanism of our body. Part of this is the lymphatic system, which is a network of vessels similar to the layout of the blood vessels in our organism. From every part of the body, toxic substances are transported via these lymphatic vessels to the smaller and larger lymph nodes, which are the 'sewage plants' of the organism. Bacteria, toxins, alien substances and waste products from the body itself (like dead cells and bacteria) are transported to these detoxification plants. Some substances, for example cows' milk and certain fats, are sent directly from the intestines, via the small lymphatic vessels situated in the intestinal wall, to the main centre of the lymphatic defence system situated in the abdomen. There, and in the various other lymph nodes, as well as the tonsils and appendix, these substances are cleaned and detoxified. After this, all waste substances that cannot be used are taken up by the venous blood and eliminated. The most important organs through which this elimination of toxins takes place are the skin, the kidneys, the lungs and the intestines. Even hundreds of years ago physicians knew that there were many interactions between the outer skin and the inner mucous membrane which could be made use of therapeutically. The spleen and the thyroid gland are also part of the defence system.

As the greatest dangers to our health develop in the abdomen, most lymphatic vessels and lymph nodes are found there. In the abdomen a very important substance for our defence, immuno globulin, is also produced. Every second, no matter how slight the danger, millions of defensive cells are used and have to be replaced over and over again.

Whenever health is at risk, the immune system will automatically react. One can understand this best by looking at simple defensive reactions that happen every day. If dust gets into the nose, we sneeze in order to get rid of it and protect our respiratory tract. If something gets into our eyes, tears will clean them. Coughing, clearing the throat and sneezing sometimes have a dual purpose: they not only help to dispose of dust particles, but also to eliminate the accumulated mucus. If we have eaten food that does not agree with us, we suffer from diarrhoea or vomiting. The main purpose of this is always the cleansing of the organism.

It is terribly important, when supplements are necessary, to detoxify the system. Nowadays I see many children with lymphatic swelling or congestion, and their systems must be cleared. I often advise parents to give their children beetroot juice, which is excellent for this purpose. Organic beetroot juice is best. Simple health problems can be cured by simple measures. With greater health problems, the organism will fight by using many different defensive measures.

There are people who have a so-called 'lymphatic constitution'. These people very often become ill when their lymphatic defences have been weakened. They then suffer from health problems, such as the common cold or a sore throat, which are nothing but a simple defence reaction of the body. Such natural reactions always have a purpose and serve to eliminate toxins. A lymphatic constitution is sometimes hereditary, but it is also possible to acquire such a constitution during the course of life. The reasons for developing a lymphatic constitution start when one is still young, for example when small children eat too many sweets or drink too much milk. In this case, the tonsils or the lymph nodes in the neck start to swell as the organism tries to neutralise the toxins. If it is not possible to neutralise all the toxins, the child may get tonsillitis (inflammation of the tonsils) and it will depend upon the physician and the parents if this inflammation is treated in the correct way by natural means, or if the child will suffer all its life from lymphatic diseases. An operation on the tonsils or treatment with antibiotics may have serious consequences, as the tonsils can no longer act as a defence organism. Then, the bronchial tubes, the mucous membranes of the sinuses and other parts of the lymphatic system will take over their defensive functions. If, in this case, the person in question eats an unhealthy diet, those secondary defensive measures will also be overstrained. Then lifelong chronic diseases of the bronchial system and the sinuses, as well as serious diseases of the abdomen, may develop.

Nowadays our immune system has to work non-stop at full power and is constantly overstressed. The cells of the immune system die by the million and cannot be replaced quickly enough. Uncountable substances alien to the human body prevent normal body functions, for any substance entering our digestive tract that cannot be used implies a loss of energy and needless work for the immune system. We are living in a world full of substances which are toxic to us, and each day many of these penetrate into our body, although most of the time such alien elements are rendered harmless by our defensive mechanism and eliminated as soon as possible.

If the medical establishment remains ignorant about these toxic substances, and if all symptoms continue to be suppressed regardless of casualties, there will be more and more chronic illness in the world. Immunity, then, is something that is very important. As I often say in lectures, children do not build up good immune systems by eating Angel Delight pudding, or a tin of tomato soup which has never seen a tomato. They need lots of fresh fruit and vegetables.

To supplement the diet, however, you could give natural chews by Nature's Best to boys and girls aged four to twelve. These are natural and delicious-tasting, and contain multivitamins and minerals to help provide nutritional help, and to act as a safeguard for children who are difficult eaters. These come in a completely natural base, which contains lecithin, acerola, lemon bioflavonoids, rutin, sunflower seeds, yeast, wheatgerm, alfalfa, papaya, date sugar, raw sugar, mannitol and fructose.

Two a day will provide your child with:

Table 4: Nutritional Content of Natural Chews

Vitamin A	4000i.u.
Vitamin D3	400i.u.
Vitamin C	60mg
Vitamin B1 (Thiamin)	2mg
Vitamin B2 (Riboflavin)	2.4mg
Vitamin B12	10mcg
Vitamin B6 (Hydrochloride)	2mg
Vitamin E	3.4i.u.
Biotin	10mcg
Nicotinamide	10mg
Pantothenic Acid	2mg
Calcium	19mg
Copper Gluconate	0.2mg
Iron	12mg
Magnesium	22mg
Choline Bitartrate	2mg
Potassium Gluconate	4mg
Inositol	2mg

Some children may need an extra vitamin B complex supplement which combines a full range of the B vitamins that are found naturally in vegetables and animal tissues, and which are essential for the health of the human body. Everyone needs a daily amount of the B complex vitamins. It is important to take B complex rather then B vitamins in isolation, because all the B vitamins work most effectively through multiple interaction with each other – for instance, a deficiency in Vitamin B2 will impair the metabolism of Vitamin B12. Also, the B vitamins are co-factors, which means they combine or work with enzymes as essential 'helper substances' within the body. Some of the B vitamins are easily destroyed by poor cooking methods or by exposure to light or air. As a result, many people who do not manage to eat regular, freshly prepared meals choose a B complex formula of vitamins and associated factors to help ensure their intake of valuable nutrients. Important functions of the B complex vitamins include:

Burning carbohydrates to release their energy
Maintaining the health of our nervous system
Assisting the metabolism of fats and proteins
Ensuring the formation of red blood cells
Helping ensure normal brain function and memory
Assisting digestion

Don't forget that vitamin C is very important if a child becomes prone to colds and flu. I prefer children to get their vitamin C from citrus fruit, red berries and blackcurrant juice. The more natural the food, the better it is for the child. As the child grows up, different nutrients may be necessary at different ages. In Table 5 I have detailed a vitamin and mineral checklist with recommended daily allowances (RDA).

Table 5: Vitamin and Mineral Checklist

Children aged 1–3

Nutrient	RDA	Nutrient	RDA
Vitamin A	400mcg	Potassium	1000mg
Vitamin D	10mcg	Calcium	800mg
Vitamin E	6mg	Phosphorus	800mg
Vitamin K	15mcg	Magnesium	80mg
Thiamin (B1)	0.7mg	Iron	10mg
Riboflavin (B2)	0.8mg	Iodine	80mcg
Niacin (B3)	9mg	Fluoride	1mg
Pantothenic acid	3mg	Zinc	10mg
Pyridoxine (B6)	1mg	Copper	0.8mg
Biotin (B8)	20mcg	Chromium	50mcg
Folic Acid	50mcg	Manganese	1.2mg
Vitamin B12	0.7mcg	Selenium	20mcg
Vitamin C	40mg	Molybdenum	40mcg

Children aged 4–6

Nutrient	RDA	Nutrient	RDA
Vitamin A	500mcg	Potassium	1400mg

Nutrient	RDA	Nutrient	RDA
Vitamin D	10mcg	Calcium	800mg
Vitamin E	7mg	Phosphorus	800mg
Vitamin K	20mcg	Magnesium	120mg
Thiamin (B1)	0.9mg	Iron	10mg
Riboflavin (B2)	1.1mg	Iodine	90mcg
Niacin (B3)	12mg	Fluoride	1.75mg
Pantothenic acid	3.5mg	Zinc	10mg
Pyridoxine (B6)	1.1mg	Copper	1.25mg
Biotin (B8)	25mcg	Chromium	90mcg
Folic Acid	75mcg	Manganese	1.75mg
Vitamin B12	1mcg	Selenium	20mcg
Vitamin C	45mg	Molybdenum	50mcg

Children aged 7–10

Nutrient	RDA	Nutrient	RDA
Vitamin A	700mcg	Potassium	1600mg
Vitamin D	10mcg	Calcium	800mg
Vitamin E	7mg	Phosphorus	800mg
Vitamin K	30mcg	Magnesium	170mg
Thiamin (B1)	1mg	Iron	10mg
Riboflavin (B2)	1.2mg	Iodine	120mcg
Niacin (B3)	13mg	Fluoride	2mg
Pantothenic acid	4.5mg	Zinc	10mg
Pyridoxine (B6)	1.4mg	Copper	1.5mg
Biotin (B8)	30mcg	Chromium	125mcg
Folic Acid	100mcg	Manganese	12.5mg
Vitamin B12	1.4mcg	Selenium	30mcg
Vitamin C	45mg	Molybdenum	100mcg

Children aged 11–14

Nutrient	RDA	Nutrient	RDA
Vitamin A	1000mcg	Potassium	200mg
Vitamin D	10mcg	Calcium	1200mg
Vitamin E	10mg	Phosphorus	1200mg
Vitamin K	45mcg	Magnesium	270mg

Thiamin (B1)	1.3mg	Iron	12mg
Riboflavin (B2)	1.5mg	Iodine	150mcg
Niacin (B3)	17mg	Fluoride	2mg
Pantothenic acid	5.5mg	Zinc	15mg
Pyridoxine (B6)	1.7mg	Copper	2mg
Biotin (B8)	76mcg	Chromium	125mcg
Folic Acid	150mcg	Manganese	3.5mg
Vitamin B12	2mcg	Selenium	40mcg
Vitamin C	50mg	Molybdenum	150mcg

Children aged 15–18

Nutrient	RDA	Nutrient	RDA
Vitamin A	1000mcg	Potassium	2000mg
Vitamin D	10mcg	Calcium	1200mg
Vitamin E	10mg	Phosphorus	1200mg
Vitamin K	65mcg	Magnesium	400mg
Thiamin (B1)	1.5mg	Iron	12mg
Riboflavin (B2)	1.8mg	Iodine	150mcg
Niacin (B3)	20mg	Fluoride	2mg
Pantothenic acid	5.5mg	Zinc	15mg
Pyridoxine (B6)	2mg	Copper	2.5mg
Biotin (B8)	70mcg	Chromium	125mcg
Folic Acid	200mcg	Manganese	3.5mg
Vitamin B12	2mcg	Selenium	50mcg
Vitamin C	60mg	Molybdenum	150mcg

Pregnant women

Nutrient	RDA	Nutrient	RDA
Vitamin A	800mcg	Potassium	2000mg
Vitamin D	10mcg	Calcium	1200mg
Vitamin E	10mg	Phosphorus	1200mg
Vitamin K	65mcg	Magnesium	320mg
Thiamin (B1)	1.5mg	Iron	30mg
Riboflavin (B2)	1.6mg	Iodine	175mcg
Niacin (B3)	17mg	Fluoride	2.5mg

Pantothenic acid	5.5mg	Zinc	15mg
Pyridoxine (B6)	2.2mg	Copper	2.5mg
Biotin (B8)	70mcg	Chromium	125mcg
Folic Acid	400mcg	Manganese	3.5mg
Vitamin B12	2.2mcg	Selenium	65mcg
Vitamin C	70mg	Molybdenum	150mcg

It is important for mothers as well as children to follow a balanced supplement programme, such as the one given in my book *Pregnancy and Childbirth*. If your child has difficulty concentrating as it grows up, extra vitamins, minerals and trace elements may be necessary; mental performance can be improved if good supplements are taken. I have had great results with supplements by Michaels, as well as enzymatic therapy and guidance on good food and supplement management, improving children's behaviour and health, and even their IQs. What is most important is that children get plenty of fresh fruit and vegetables and, when necessary, supplements.

I must, however, advise caution when giving your child supplements. If these are overdone it can lead to problems, so please take professional advice and guidance to ensure that the child is not ingesting larger amounts of nutrients than necessary when taking supplements.

THIRTEEN

Organic or Regular?

When I go to supermarkets these days it is with the greatest pleasure that I see the organic sections growing and growing. Let's be honest, organic food tastes a lot better, smells a lot better and has the vitamins, minerals and trace elements that our bodies really need. Unfortunately, it is not easy to grow organic food in today's society and a lot more effort is needed to encourage more people to eat it. If everyone ate organic food, it would not be as expensive; people often tell me that buying such food is a problem due to the cost. More promotion must be done to increase the demand for organically grown food, which would then increase consumption, allowing prices to fall.

There is no doubt that when people have degenerative diseases, their health improves when they change over to organic food and beverages. I have seen this in many of my patients, and with some degenerative diseases the problem is completely overcome. I put great emphasis on eating organic food as much as possible. The evidence is there that this is a tremendous plus point for health.

Up to the age of five in particular, it is extremely important that the child eats the very best. If a child's appetite is poor, give it some *Centaurium* (three or four drops twice a day). I am often asked how to make nice dishes with organic food for a children's party. I find that this is an excellent opportunity to introduce children to natural foods –a 'natural foods tasting party' can be really fun. Look at sunflower seeds and how much you can do with them – they are delicious toasted. Experiment with dried fruits and special bread, and specially made sugar-free sweets and chocolates (available from health-food shops), all of which can be made very appealing to children, even for a party, and are healthy, natural foods. There are plenty of good cookery books that will give you all kinds of ideas.

For pregnant and lactating women, it is important to eat foods that have all the necessary vitamins and minerals in them. This is also important for children when they are growing up, and especially for teenagers, as the adolescent growth spurt is a time of enormous nutritional demand. As children grow up and there are more demands on them to study, they often need good organic food to help them through this period, just as they did when they were babies after being weaned onto solid foods. Good food is necessary for physical development, but there is no need to push children – they will determine which foods they like and dislike. It is just a matter of getting your child used to foods that are important for its health. I usually advise training children in their first year to enjoy healthy foods. As they grow up, their preference will be for nutritious foods.

It is quite interesting to see the increasing importance placed on cereals, and especially organically grown grains, in society today. I have already discussed cereals and whole grains, but I would like to expand a little on this subject as it is so important. There are some very good recipes that can be used to encourage children to eat muesli, which is very nutritious. Mixed with half a banana, orange juice and a grated apple, muesli will give a child all the vitamins, minerals and trace elements it needs, as well as busy mothers, who need a good breakfast, which is the most important meal of the day.

Not only are cereals the staple diet of many nations and ethnic groups, but raw or cooked cereals were used in the past to heal many different diseases. At the beginning of the 20th century, raw, freshly ground cereals like the mueslis of Prof. Kollath, Dr Bruker and Dr Max Bircher-Benner were very popular. Thousands of patients in the Bircher-Benner clinic in Zurich and in Dr Bruker's clinic in Germany were cured of serious chronic diseases. Bircher muesli is still so well known in Switzerland that 65 per cent of the Swiss eat it almost every day for breakfast. There is a wide selection of ready-made muesli in every health shop and even in supermarkets there, and this is also the case in Germany and other European countries. However, while most people think it is good for their health to eat ready-made muesli, it cannot be compared with the benefits of home-made muesli. Of course, it is still better to eat ready-made muesli than white rolls with jam.

The difference between Kollath, Bruker and Bircher muesli is that the first two mueslis consist mainly of different types of cereal, which constitute their most important ingredients. Bircher muesli, however, contains very little cereal and the most important ingredient is apple. These different types of muesli all have great healing powers and it is surprising how many illnesses are relieved when people eat them for a period of time.

KOLLATH'S ORIGINAL MUESLI RECIPE

Serves one person.

Ingredients:
75g non-sticky (without much gluten) wheat, rye or barley
100g water
A little cream/buttermilk
Finely chopped fruit of your choice

Method:
At night, grind the wheat, rye or barley, or a mixture of the three, in a coffee grinder. Mix this with the water, stir well and leave to soak overnight. In the morning, add a little more water (if needed) and mix the porridge with a little cream or buttermilk (made from raw milk). Then add some fruit. This porridge can also be prepared with a little salt, herbs, natural spices, flavours, tomatoes, etc. It all depends on your taste, and at what time of the day you like to eat it.

BIRCHER'S ORIGINAL MUESLI RECIPE

Ingredients:
8g wholegrain wheat
1 teaspoon lemon juice

1 dessertspoon cream
200g apples
1 dessertspoon grated nuts or almonds

Put the wheat through a shredder or grain mill. Then mix the shredded grain with a little water and let it soak overnight. In the morning, stir the lemon juice and cream into the porridge. Then wash and dry the apples and grate them, and stir immediately into the mixture. Sprinkle the nuts over the porridge before serving.

Originally, Dr Bircher-Benner used condensed milk instead of fresh cream because dairy products at that time were not treated very hygienically and condensed milk seemed to be the best choice. Nowadays, it is better to use fresh cream. Even most people who are allergic to milk products can digest this, because milk fat is always easier to digest than milk protein or milk sugar. For people who can digest raw food without problems, Bircher muesli is a very healthy dish indeed. You can make it even tastier by adding, for example, one or two other kinds of fruit, sunflower seeds, sesame seeds, pine nuts, different kinds of dried fruits etc.

If you are not as healthy as you would wish, you should eat as simply as possible, only using fresh ingredients. Every addition uses up extra energy for digestion and you will need every bit of energy for healing. For this reason, fasting is a wonderful healer. When you are fasting, no energy is lost by the digestion of food and the body can heal itself.

If you cannot digest raw food, do not eat it! If you suffer from intestinal or stomach problems, you should first cure your disease before you eat muesli or similar foods. The best treatment for all these diseases is to eat only cereal jelly for a few days, weeks or even longer, and you can make this at home.

PREPARATION OF CEREAL JELLY
Wholegrain cereal should be ground and soaked overnight (every household should possess a grinder). The next day, these grains should be cooked slowly for at least an hour and then passed through a sieve.

You can season this with a little sea salt or herbs or, if you prefer the jelly to be sweet, add a little natural honey or pure maple syrup, or Stevia (a natural sweetener from plants which the Native American Indians used).

If you suffer from gastroenteritis, or other stomach or intestinal problems, you should eat as much jelly as you like three or four times a day and nothing else. If these health problems have passed, you can try to eat the softly cooked whole grains; chew them thoroughly and for a long time. While you are eating this diet, the stomach wall and the wall of the intestines will be covered with a layer of jelly which will give the body a chance to heal. Between these jelly meals, you should only drink water or herbal teas.

In the beginning, you can use oats, wheat or barley and, later on, other cereals. You will discover what helps you most. Then you can start gradually eating other foods, such as cereal soup, boiled potatoes and vegetables which are easy to digest and do not produce wind.

When all your health problems have gone, you can gradually introduce some raw food (like carrots or fennel). To start with, only have a teaspoonful at a time and then slowly increase the quantity. After about three weeks you may try to eat some muesli. However, if you begin to feel ill again, go back to phase one and start all over again, eating only cereal jelly.

While dieting like this, natural and homoeopathic medicaments will support the treatment. Please be patient, because this is the only way if you really want to cure a serious illness of the intestines. It all depends on you, on your intelligence, understanding and willpower.

LACTIC ACID

It is dangerous to your health when your body contains too much acid as a consequence of our modern diets. On the other hand, there is one kind of acid which is not only harmless, but which our organism needs in order to function properly. This is lactic acid, and it contains very special bacteria that fulfil many important tasks in our body. Amongst other things, it produces several vitamins (like vitamin B12) and it is part of the defence system of our body. In our skin and in the mucous membranes, this acid forms a protective coating and also helps with the digestion of proteins and stimulates bowel movement.

Concentrated lactic acid is used for the treatment of serious intestinal diseases, like dysentery, typhoid and cholera.

The beneficial kind of lactic acid can only be found in milk or dairy products when these have been made from raw, completely natural milk. You will find the right kind of lactic acid in products like kefir, buttermilk and whey made from raw milk.

Yoghurt, which is very popular, very seldom contains the kind of lactic acid our body needs. There also is a danger that, with regular yoghurt consumption, abnormal bacterial flora will develop, whereby the body's own intestinal bacteria is slowly replaced by yoghurt bacteria (see Hans-Peter Rusch). This can be quite dangerous for our general health.

Better suppliers of lactic acid are vegetables from bio-dynamic cultivation like, for example, sauerkraut (pickled cabbage), carrots etc. Raw sauerkraut is easier to digest than cooked sauerkraut and, when both kinds are mixed together, it tastes better. Whey (available in health food shops) and cottage cheese are usually wonderful sources of lactic acid, and even people with a milk allergy can often digest them.

A small glass of whey or sauerkraut juice before a meal is good for digestion. Regular consumption of whey or lactic acid vegetables will immensely enhance the body's own defence system.

DR KUHL'S LACTIC ACID MUESLI
The healing properties of this preparation are even greater than any of the mueslis described previously, because the ingredients are prepared on the basis of lactic acid fermentation. During this preparation, many enzymes, vitamins, hormones, natural aromatic substances and natural antibiotics are developed.

This muesli should not be eaten daily. I recommend it as a remedy and should be prepared only once in a while, when you are feeling overtired, overworked or depressed, lacking in energy and susceptible to infections.

Mix roughly ground cereal with 30 per cent of water and then knead thoroughly by hand on a wooden board and form into a ball. Leave this ball uncovered in a clean dish, in a warm, humid place, for 24 hours. After this time, you will find that the mixture has become rather humid and sticky: when you press it together with one hand, it sticks together, but when you open your hand, it crumbles apart. Shape it into a ball again and leave it untouched for four days.

On the morning of the fifth day, it should be made into porridge with some buttermilk or whey, and then eaten for breakfast with a little honey. This preparation should always be done as described here; only in this way can all the vital substances develop. Be careful not to eat the muesli if it starts smelling bad.

THE WRONG KIND OF FOOD

Did you realise that in the past 100–150 years eating habits in Western industrialised countries have changed more than in the previous 5,000–6,000 years? Food which at one time was very expensive became cheaper, and at last most people could afford to buy meat, fruit and sweets and eat their fill. Today, in Europe and the USA, we live in a time of abundance never before known. In fact, in this part of the world there is more food available than people need, but are we any healthier because of this? No – quite the contrary! Never before have so many people been chronically ill. The food we eat no longer contains the nutrients necessary for the correct functioning of our digestive systems, and therefore most of our diseases are caused by, and start with, metabolic disorders.

Most of us eat far too much and, due to the over-consumption of denatured food and a lack of exercise and fresh air, many people – especially in the latter part of their lives – become caricatures of themselves. The Grecian ideal of a beautiful human being no longer seems to exist. Nowadays we rarely see a really beautiful and healthy-looking person. Most of us are comfort-loving gourmets or gourmands, and either too fat or too thin. Our legs are swollen, our feet flat, our backs bent, our necks stiff. We lose our hair, suffer from dental decay, headaches, flatulence, constipation and depression. We tire easily and, worst of all, many of us no longer enjoy life. Many people never feel really well.

Maybe you think I am exaggerating, since most people we know seem to be quite healthy, with the exception of some elderly people who suffer from old-age diseases. This, of course, we consider as being completely normal. Certainly, most people *seem* to be healthy.

However, when you get to know them really well, you can often be surprised. Even your best friend or business partner, whom you see almost daily, might suffer from chronic health problems you never suspected.

It should never be thought normal when elderly people are ill, although even some patients themselves tend to think in this way. Such thoughts are very alarming and completely wrong. An Austrian newspaper, *The Kurier*, stated on 15 May 1997: 'More and more young people enjoy poor health. Over two million Austrians feel physically impaired. This tendency among young people is increasing. About 30 per cent of all Austrians are physically affected in their daily lives.'

This shows that even the younger generation is not as healthy as it was in the past. Austria is not the only country with such problems. More and more people in our industrialised countries suffer from chronic diseases, and others who think they are healthy should take another look at themselves.

Nowadays, people seem to think that dental decay, headaches, allergies and other such ailments are normal and that one 'just has to live with' these problems. This idea is nonsense! It is so important that both mothers and children take care of their health.

HEALTH PROBLEMS ALWAYS HAVE A REASON
When the human organism goes on strike and does not function correctly, there must be a reason for it. Our organism is a kind of living machine which, like any other machine, needs a specific type of fuel. Apart from oxygen and water, our most important fuel is nutrition. Even before we are born, our body was built with the help of this fuel. Therefore it is very important that a future mother should eat healthy food as this builds up the fundamental framework of the body and the mind of her child.

The foundation of any building must be firm and should be built only with top quality materials. Likewise, a healthy body should be built and maintained only with first-class food. All other factors, even if they seem to be elemental, are of secondary importance. No disease can be healed, even with the best medicine, if one does not eat a healthy diet.

INDUSTRIAL ADULTERATION OF OUR FOOD

Our organism adapted itself to the life and the eating habits of the first primitive people during its original evolution. Since then, as long as human nutrition did not change too much, then the assimilation, transformation and utilisation of food was never much of a problem for our digestive organs. However, in the course of time, human nutritional habits changed in many ways. There were migrations of people to other continents where the food was completely different. Sometimes it was very difficult and took quite some time for their digestive organs to adapt to a new kind of nutrition. But as the food was still completely natural and contained most of the nutrients the human body needed, after some time the organism adjusted itself quite well.

Unfortunately, during the last 100–150 years, the situation has changed increasingly in the negative sense. Now the chances of the survival of the human race do not depend primarily upon nuclear danger, but on the degeneration and chronic diseases caused mainly by the malnutrition from which the inhabitants of the industrialised countries suffer. Much of the food we eat today is completely incompatible with our digestive system.

For our body, the assimilation and transformation of this so-called 'food' is extremely difficult. Whereas in prehistoric times all food was 100 per cent natural, today 80 per cent of our modern food has been adulterated to such an extent that it contains hardly any vitamins, minerals or other vital substances. It does, however, contain calories!

Our food still contains proteins, carbohydrates and fats, which unfortunately have been modified in many ways. Most of this food has been overheated, pressed, cooled, tumbled, frozen or defrosted, and during every one of these procedures, vital nutrients are lost and countless additives are used to replace them.

'New' foods are invented all the time, and colourings and uncountable other substances are used to enhance the taste and the appearance of the food, and make everything we eat still more attractive. The consumer often has no idea what he or she is actually eating. During the process of refining our food, manufacturers use up to 3,500 chemical additives. Quite a few of these additives may be harmful or even poisonous for the human organism, but as long as this has not been proved absolutely, the food can still be sold.

Most people believe that the quantities of these substances used for the 'refining' of our food are so small that they can do no harm. Also, those responsible for our health do not seem to know that many such substances could have a toxic or even lethal effect, even when diluted a hundred or a thousand times. Of course, the defence mechanisms of our body are able to render many of these toxins harmless. However, any person who consumes the same foods or soft drinks over a long period will finally accumulate so many harmful substances in his or her body that he or she will no longer be able to eliminate these.

FAST FOODS AND MODERN DRINKS

In the last century, we seem to have forgotten which foods are really suitable for us. Children eat sweets and drink cola and parents wonder why their 'little darlings' are so restless or look so pale. The whole of the body, including the nervous system and the brain, are receiving artificial substitutes instead of the needed nutrients. Fast food and ready-made meals – which have no nutritional value – have become bestsellers. We have less work in the kitchen now; we only have to add a little water to some of these dishes and put them in the microwave oven and they are ready to eat. Soup, gravies and sauces which contain nothing but salt, flavourings and other chemical ingredients do not deserve to be called 'natural'. We are so used to products such as potato chips, crisps and all kinds of other snacks that we no longer think of them as harmful. We may be used to this food, but our organism will never get used to it!

During all the processing such food goes through, most of its vital nutrients are destroyed and therefore the manufacturers think it a good idea to add minute quantities of synthetic vitamins and minerals. Although insignificant, these quantities may then be printed on the label along with the other ingredients. In my opinion, this is fraud. One cannot take away almost all of the valuable nutrients and then replace them with artificially made substances. The chemical formula may be correct, but these substances can never be compared to natural vitamins and minerals, which cannot be reproduced in a factory. They lack vitality and life.

Modern drinks are just as bad, or even worse. In former days, people drank only water or sometimes, as an exception, a little beer or wine which was diluted with water. When very thirsty, people drank water mixed with a little vinegar. In modern society, people drink more and more alcohol and this tendency continues to rise. Many children and adults drink 'soft drinks' instead of water. The consumption of these drinks is estimated as being an average of 130 litres per person annually. In North America, this figure is even higher. Most of these drinks contain an excess of sugar and additives, as well as many calories, which spoil a healthy appetite. Many people have developed an addiction to coffee and cola drinks. These problems were discussed in detail earlier in this book, but because of their importance, I cannot stress the points I have made strongly enough.

GENETIC FACTORS
You might begin to ask, 'What about genes? We read that "bad" genes are the cause of many diseases.' Let me try to answer this question in a simple way. Genes are 'in'. Many scientific and non-scientific people are very enthusiastic about genetic engineering. They believe that this will cure or prevent many diseases. Let us hope they are right, but let me remind you that in the beginning, people were just as delighted with the discovery of sulpha-drugs or antibiotics.

Genes are certainly part of the foundations of the body. Inside a living cell, a gene is like a commanding officer, like a general in the army or the captain of a ship. There are good and bad captains, just as there are good and bad genes. Good genes bring health and bad genes can be the cause of certain (sometimes dangerous) diseases.

If the leadership of a captain is not satisfactory, the company will try to find a replacement. So, for many years scientists have been dreaming of the possibility of exchanging bad genes for good ones. By doing so, scientists hope to rescue humanity from some terrible diseases – a wonderful and noble thought!

Until some time ago this seemed to be nothing more than wishful thinking, but quite recently modern science has made so much progress that this idea is no longer an impossible dream. Not only in the case of plants or animals, but also in the case of human beings, certain genes in our cells can now be replaced. However, we should realise that the human cell is a very complicated entity, a microcosm. This microcosm consists of an uncountable number of components, which are solid, liquid or gaseous. Also, it is known that the entire cell-life is being influenced by many different energy flows and that even our mental attitude and thoughts influence internal functions and our state of health. Every fraction of a second many different actions and reactions – about which we still know very little – take place inside our cells.

In my opinion, most scientists still see the human body as a kind of machine and because of this they believe that, like a machine, it would be a good idea to exchange the bad parts in a human being for good parts. However, the human body is a living entity. Within the millions of cells in our body, all the different components, actions and reactions are in every respect completely interdependent on one another.

Also, cells containing bad genes which, under certain circumstances, may provoke disease, are living entities that fulfil certain specific tasks. In all our body cells, all the components collaborate in order to render the cell functional. As long as the person concerned keeps a healthy lifestyle and eats the right food, and if there are no extremely harmful influences, most negative genetic factors remain 'latent' (dormant) and will not cause any damage. Certain babies may never suffer from diseases for which they were predestined because of bad genes. However, if, for example, their mothers smoke or drink during pregnancy, or if as they grow up these children live an unhealthy life, some of the disease-provoking bad genes in their cells may get out of hand and become active.

Of course, it seems to be an excellent idea, if it is possible, to prevent the development of MS, diabetes or any other serious disease which may have dire consequences for the person in question or his or her offspring. As I said before, in a living cell all the components are closely related and dependent on one another. When the genes in a cell, which up to that moment were closely connected with all the other components of that cell, are exchanged for new genes, all of the former relationships within the cell are broken up. Now, every part of the cell and all the different energies will have to adjust to the requirements and the wavelength of the new genes. We do not know if this will be possible, and we do not know what the consequences will be.

However, under the constant pressure of pharmaceutical companies, which see the development of genetic engineering as one of the great money-makers of the future, scientists compete with one another in order to win the race. I wonder what the future will bring – but we should be prepared for some very disagreeable surprises.

The best way in which you can prevent disease is to live in such a way that you will build up a strong resistance, so that your defence system will always function in an optimal way.

FOOD THROUGH THE AGES

Coming to the end of this book, I remember how in many of the countries Dr Vogel and I visited together, there wasn't the hygiene we were used to in Europe. In primeval times, people were used to this. Many years ago, at school, I learned about the living and eating habits of primitive people. When we were small, my friends and I were fascinated by the adventurous lives of these brave people who, after hunting all day long, sat around their fires at night, eating the meat and chewing the bones of the animals they had slaughtered. Even today, many of my patients believe that eating meat two or even three times a day will not cause harm to the human body as it has been used to the digestion of great quantities of meat for thousands of years. However, they couldn't be more wrong. Much of what we learned in our youth came from the romantic imaginations of fertile minds. Now, thanks to the newest methods of excavation and analysis, we know that for a very long time in the history of man, the hunting of wild animals was very difficult and dangerous, and people hardly ate any meat at all. By analysing the stomach contents of primitive people (which have been preserved in ice or layers of the earth), we have learned much more about them. The first people who lived in the forests of Africa ate roots, grass, tubers, bulbs, fresh sprouts and shoots, fruit, mushrooms and anything else which nature provided. They also ate birds' eggs, worms and insects, but were mainly vegetarian.

During many thousands of years, the human body became adapted to processing the natural food which was available and its organs and digestive system have developed accordingly. Since then, our digestive system still functions in the same way. We know now that even the smallest changes in the construction of an organ will take hundreds of years and, in those times, the heart, the lungs, the kidneys and most of the other parts of the body were already the same as ours are today. Biological structures were gradually formed so that they could fulfil their different functions. All the useful nutrients which primeval food contained were assimilated and used by the organism. The food of former times was very hard, tough and fibrous and had to be chewed over and over again. For this reason, our ancestors' teeth and jaws were much stronger and healthier than ours are today, enabling them to cope with the food available to them at that time.

THE AGE OF NEANDERTHAL MAN
About 50,000 years ago, Neanderthal Man discovered fire and gradually learned how to roast meat. From time to time, he managed to hunt large animals by using sticks and stones, but this was always very dangerous and exhausting. The meat was then eaten exclusively by men, who believed that by eating part of a strong and dangerous animal they would inherit its characteristics. It is very interesting that, even today, there are people who believe this and many, even seriously ill people, are inclined to think that, without eating meat, they will lose their strength.

As a matter of fact, the major part of the daily food of primitive people consisted of wild vegetables, fruit and anything else edible that the women could find. Even today primitive people leave the work to the women – the men prefer to hunt or to sit in the sun. After some months or years, when their food sources became scarce, they started to explore further afield. For a long time these primitive people, because of their eating habits, were forced to live as nomads, but after they had learned to cultivate the soil, they gradually settled down in one place.

Although now life became easier for them and they themselves could cultivate many different plants, these cultivated plants contained only a fraction of the vital components found in naturally growing plants or in the other food which the women gathered while people were still living as nomads. Long ago, the first people usually had a wide choice of hundreds of different plants. Later, when they settled down, their choice became quite limited and, especially in the beginning of that period, their food no longer contained all the nutrients that they had been used to and needed for their health. While learning more about land cultivation even later on, the choice of food became much greater and deficiency symptoms, from which some of the people had been suffering, disappeared.

FURTHER DEVELOPMENTS

About 6,000 years ago, the Egyptians planted the first cereals, beans and many kinds of vegetables. With goats, sheep and donkeys, simple stockbreeding began. Meat was available only when an animal had to be slaughtered and was always regarded as a luxury. As an alternative, people occasionally ate fish or small game.

The main meal always consisted of gruel or porridge prepared with coarsely ground cereals, and was eaten with beans, onions and other vegetables. By mixing this flour with water and allowing it to dry on stones in the sun, this cereal was used to make simple flat cakes, which provided some variety. These flat cakes, which people still eat in Egypt and some other countries, were made from thin layers of unfermented dough and baked in the sun. Later, such cakes were baked in the oven, very much like the Mexican enchiladas and tacos, Scandinavian knäckebrot or Italian polenta. People drank water, or water mixed with a little vinegar (which was made from fermented fruit). This was an excellent thirst quencher and was also used as a remedy for some health problems. The Egyptians knew how to brew a simple kind of beer, while dates and other fruits were appreciated as sweets.

In the course of time, as agriculture and stockbreeding developed more fully, there was a wider choice of foods, but cereals became more important and remained the principal food in many countries throughout the Middle Ages, and almost up to the present time. Most people were poor and could afford only the bare necessities of life. They worked many hours a day and were obliged to give the greater part of their harvest to the big landowners. With the exception of Sundays and special holidays, they ate no meat. Most of their food was hard and full of fibre, but by eating this simple food, working hard and being outside in the fresh air most of the day, these people were rarely ill.

Wholemeal cereals are extremely healthy. They disperse their regenerative nutrients to every part of the body. It is even better to combine cereals with vegetables, as these increase their nutritional value even more. The combination of different raw and cooked vegetables, as was customary in olden times, is excellent. Raw, whole cereal grains are a living food as, even after thousands of years – if stored correctly – they can still germinate. For around 6,000 years, people mainly ate oats, corn, millet, buckwheat and other cereals. After the harvest, the grains were dried a little and then beaten in such a way that the husk was gradually separated from the corn and could be passed through a sieve. During this process the cornstarch changed into a kind of sugar, which still contained all the valuable nutrients. By mixing the coarse flour with water, it was made into gruel or porridge, which, without being cooked, had a sweet and succulent taste.

Cereals are an excellent food for mankind as they contain carbohydrates, protein and fat, as well as vitamins, minerals and many other vital elements in the right proportions. Wholemeal cereals are a natural and nourishing food which is also inexpensive and very resistant to decay. Each kind of cereal has its own characteristics and contains different nutrients, which are dependent on the climate and the properties of the soil. Rice is the most popular cereal in the East, while corn is the most important cereal in the West. Oats are eaten mostly in the polar latitudes, while millet is the main cereal of Africa and the grasslands. The people of Central Europe have always had a preference for wheat, rye and barley.

In former times, everybody used freshly ground cereals or chewed the roasted grains, sometimes adding a little salt to make them really tasty. The food of the Roman army consisted of a daily ration of 750g wholegrain wheat or barley. In every cohort (a Roman army unit) the soldiers carried a mill for grinding these grains. A third of these were eaten as gruel and the rest was made into flat cakes, which could be eaten while the soldiers were marching. As additional food, they also ate vegetables and fruit that they 'found' during their military campaigns. Consequently, these soldiers were very healthy and became famous for their stamina.

In the beginning, when cereals were ground, the result was a mixture of fine and rough substances. This was good for the teeth and the digestive system. The Greeks, as well as the Romans, all ate barley and wheat but as civilisation developed and more people moved into the towns, nutritional habits changed. Barley became the food of the poor people and the army, but the rich, upper classes preferred to eat wheat. Wheat is easily digested and much appreciated because of the many ways in which it can be used. It permits the production of the finest flour, which makes refined and exquisite pastry.

In Roman times, the lifestyle of the rich, upper classes was very decadent. At the many festive occasions to which hundreds of guests were invited, they ate abundant meals that consisted of many courses and exotic dishes. Vast quantities of meat, venison and poultry were eaten, and there was no shortage of wine and other drinks. At that time, wine was diluted with water, as undiluted wine was considered to be a drink for 'barbarians'. Such rich meals were considered a status symbol and were a sign of class-consciousness. Many members of the upper classes suffered from gluttony and often became chronically ill. As in the decadent times of the Greeks and Romans, today most people prefer to eat wheat and fail to realise that any kind of refined flour is a 'vitamin and mineral robber', as is our refined white sugar. It is no surprise, then, that in those ancient times, the rich, upper classes suffered from diseases similar to those we know today.

Today, I am happy to be living in a knowledgeable society. I see the rapid changes in the development of health, which may even be accelerating too quickly, as we belong to nature and we have to obey the laws of nature. We may be able to clone, but nature will still take its course and unless we let this happen and give nature its rightful place, then our system will fall apart.

FOURTEEN

Conclusion

It is a wonderful privilege to be a father. It is an even greater privilege to be a grandfather and to understand a little more about children's behaviour, to realise that in this very permissive world one can set a good example and make children feel secure by letting them know that you are there for them. Everybody in life has a function, and a mother's relationship to her child is probably the most perfect one. They know each other. They may even know what the other is thinking. The relationship between mother and child is one of the most precious possessions on this earth. One can never underestimate the value of it.

It is important to learn to allow your children to lead their own lives, while at the same time letting them know that you are there for them. My mother always told me about her grandmother and what a wonderful part she played in her life. Her children and grandchildren loved her so much that they talked about her almost daily because they felt a fantastic security knowing she was there for them. My mother's other grandmother made life such a misery for her own children and grandchildren that, on the day she died, they were all happy that she had gone. Although they all tried to help her, she refused all help offered and chose to live life as a recluse, having nothing to do with her children or grandchildren. What a very sad existence. Whenever my mother, aunts and uncles spoke fondly of their mother and grandmother, I always had a great desire to be like them for my own children and, even today, I continue to strive to achieve this.

When I think of the tremendous influence that love can have on the life of a family and what it can lead to, I recall my mother's eldest brother who was a military officer. During the invasion of Holland, he met a German general who revealed the love he had for my grandmother long before the war. Because of that, many lives were saved when he contacted my uncle, enabling him to save his people. This was a reward for the love that my grandmother had for him when he was young and still impressionable.

In the world today, where everything is becoming more economically geared, we must not forget that love still has the strongest power to save this world from destruction. If everyone could develop the kind of love that a mother has for her child when bringing him or her into this world, we might have a better society. The relationship of mother and child, which can, and should, be perfect, might show us all the way to make the world a better place.

Endnotes

1   Terry Burnham & Jay Phelan, *Mean Genes: From Sex to Money to Food: Taming Our Primal Instincts* (Simon & Schuster, London, 2000), pp. 59–82.

2   University of Sunderland Autism Research Unit (www.osiris.sunderland.ac.uk).

3   S.O. Shaheen *et al.* 'Measles and Atopy in Guinea-Missau', *The Lancet* (1996), 347 (28), pp. 1,792–1,796.

4   National Asthma Campaign (www.asthma.org.uk) fact sheet, audit 1997/98.

5   National Asthma Campaign press release, audit 2001

6   G. Rook, 'Give Us This Day Our Daily Germs', *Immunology Today* (1998), 19 (3), pp. 113–16

7   'When Should a Child be Immunised?' Department of Health website, www.immunisation.org.uk

8   D. Vison, 'Immunisation Does Not Rule Out Tetanus', letter published in *British Medical Journal* (2000), 320, p.383

9   A. Wakefield, 'Lieal-lymphoid-nodular Hyperplasia, Non-specific Colitis and Pervasive Development Disorder in Children', *The Lancet* (1998), 351 (28), pp. 637–41.

10 Website relating to MMR immunisation and autism, www.autism.com

11 Dr Bernard Rimland, quoted in the *Daily Mail*, Tuesday, 12 August 1999, p. 5.

12 JABS website, www.jabs.org.uk

13 'Admission on Gulf War Spurs Debate on Medical Records', *Nature*
    (1997), 390 (6), pp. 3–4.

14 G. Rook, 'Gulf War Syndrome: Is It Due to a Systematic Shift in
    Cytokine Balance towards a Th2 Profile?', *The Lancet* (1997), 349,
    pp. 1,831–1,833.

Appendix: Useful Addresses

The Informed Parent
PO Box 870
Harrow
Middlesex
HA3 7UW
0208 8611022

JABS
1 Gawsworth Road
Golborne
Warrington
WA3 3RF
01942 713565

Hadley Wood Healthcare
28 Crescent West
Hadley West
Barnet
Herts
EN4 0EJ
0208 4418352

Nature's Best
PO Box 1
Tunbridge Wells

Primal Health Research
(Published quarterly by Dr
  Odent)
59 Roderick Road
London
NW3 2NP
0207 2675123

Society of Homoeopaths
2 Artizans Road
Northampton
NN1 4HU
01604 621400

Auchenkyle
South Woods
Troon
Ayrshire
KA10 7EL
Jan de Vries Helpline:
  01292 318846

Bibliography

1. *The Need of Children*, Mia Kellmer Pringle (Hutchinson, London).
2. *Improve your Child's IQ and Behaviour*, Dr Stephen Schoenthaler (BBC Books, London).
3. *Positive Parent Power*, Helen Bethune (Thorsons Publishing, London).
4. *Sharing Nature with Children*, Joseph Cornell (Dawn Publishing, Nevada City, USA).
5. *Brain Injury*, Ian Hunter (Ashgrove Press, Bath, UK).
6. *Is This Your Child?*, Doris Rapp, MD Quill (William Morrow, New York, USA).
7. *Nanny Knows Best*, Nanny Smith and Nina Grunfeld (BBC Series, London).
8. *Your Second Baby*, Patricia Hewitt and Wendy Rose Neill (Thorsons Publishing, London).
9. *If You Love Me, Don't Feed Me Junk*, Sandy Gooch (Reston Publishing Co., Reston, Virginia).
10. *Healing Touch*, Maria and Marcus Webb (Godsfield Books, London)

Index